FENG'S WAY:
TO PERMANENT WEIGHT LOSS FOR ADULTS AND CHILDREN

BREAKTHROUGH IN NATURAL WEIGHT LOSS

By

SIMON FENG, M.D.

© 2004 by SIMON FENG, M.D. All rights reserved.

No part of this book may be reproduced, stored in a retrieval system, or transmitted by any means, electronic, mechanical, photocopying, recording, or otherwise, without written permission from the author.

ISBN: 1-4140-4704-5 (e-book)
ISBN: 1-4140-4705-3 (Paperback)

Library of Congress Control Number: 2003099539

This book is printed on acid-free paper.

Printed in the United States of America
Bloomington, IN

1stBooks - rev. 01/29/04

Acknowledgements:

Many people deserve my deep appreciation. The final form that this book takes was greatly influenced by their input. My thanks go to my brother, Dr. Franc Feng, for his initial direction and critique, as well as instruction on using Word. I also wish to thank my mother, Mrs. Catherine Feng, for her years of nurturing. I would like to acknowledge my gratitude to my mother-in-law, Barbara Fysh, for her input and excellent editing. My toughest critic, and therefore my most valuable critic, was of course my wife Wendy, who is also my strongest supporter. Lastly, I must not neglect to extend my gratitude to Sally Sturgell, the dedicated librarian at Johnson Memorial Hospital, whose help has been invaluable.

The advice given in this book is based upon research and observations by the author. It is not meant to replace the medical advice from your personal physician.

For my wife, Wendy, my children, George and William, and in Memory of my Father

TABLE OF CONTENTS

PREFACE: FENG'S WAY TO PERMANENT WEIGHT LOSS FOR ADULTS AND CHILDREN XI
    A Socio-Cultural Approach xi

SECTION ONE   THE PROBLEM 1

CHAPTER ONE: THE GOAL 3
    Permanent Weight Loss 3
    The Law of Conservation of Energy 5
    The Problem with Diets 9
    How about Exercise? 10
    Cures vs. Controls 11

CHAPTER TWO: THE EPIDEMIC OF OBESITY 15
    The Scope of the Problem 15
    Prevalence of Obesity (Maps) 17
    Why this Epidemic is Silent 20
    What Can Be Done? 21

SECTION TWO   CURRENT TREATMENT PHILOSOPHIES 23

CHAPTER THREE: HERBAL WEIGHT LOSS AND NATURAL DIETARY SUPPLEMENTS 25
    Popularity of Herbal/Nutritional Supplements 25
    Myths and Misconceptions about Herbal Remedies in General 26
        Myth #1. Herbal medicines are safer than conventional medications. 26
        Myth #2. Herbal medicines are natural 28
        Myth #3. Herbal medicines are standardized. 29
        Myth #4. Herbal medications have little or no side effects 30
        Myth #5. Herbal medicine is more trustworthy than traditional medicine 31
        Myth #6. Herbal medications are backed up by research 33

    Nutritional Supplements / Herbal Medications and the FDA 34
    Herbal Remedies in General 35
    Herbal Weight Loss 37
    Metabolism Boosters 37
CHAPTER FOUR: THE MEDICAL MODEL OF OBESITY 39
    Obesity as a Disease 39
    Medical Treatment of Obesity 40
    Full-Service and Self-Service Medical Care 40
    Currently Available Pharmaceutical Treatments 41
    Metabolic and Genetic Components of Obesity 43
    Short Comings of the Medical Model 46
    Bariatric Surgery 47
CHAPTER FIVE: MEDICAL REASONS FOR WEIGHT GAIN 51
    Hypothyroidism 51
    Cushing's Syndrome 51
    Post-Partum Weight Gain 52
    Chronic Fatigue 53
    Sleep Apnea 54
    Effects of Medications 55
    Smoking Cessation 55
    Serious Illness 56
    Summary 57

SECTION THREE A NEW VIEWPOINT 59
CHAPTER SIX: UNHEALTHY ATTITUDES 61
    The Sociological/Cultural Basis of Obesity 62
    Changes in Social Structure 62
    Changes in the Content of the Modern Diet 63
    More Sedentary Lifestyle 64
    Changes in Ideal Body Image 65
    Unhealthy Attitudes 66
        Aversion to Wasting Food 66
        Quantumization of Food 67

  Unhealthy Attitudes are Learned in Childhood 68
  Food as Reward/Entitlement 69
  Food as a Surrogate for Love 71
  Food to Make Up For Feelings of Inadequacy 71
 Gender Differences in Attitudes Toward Food 72
 Socioeconomic Differences in Attitudes Toward Food 72
 The Diet Mentality 73
 Why I Do Not Believe In Calorie Counting or Target Weights 74
 Key Differences Between Overweight and Normal Weight People 75
 The Sociological Inertia of Culture 77

CHAPTER SEVEN: UNHEALTHY EATING PATTERNS **79**
 Non-Wasters of Food 80
 Food as Entertainment 84
 Avoidance of Public Eating / Meal Skippers 87
 The Grazer 89
 The Sweet Tooth 91
 Liquid Calories 92
 Comfort Eating 94
 Binge Eating 98
 Dieting 99
 Eating out of Boredom/ Eating to Stay Awake 100
 How We Become Overweight 102
 Natural Weight Loss Through Normal Eating 103
 What Then Is Normal? 104
 Eating Patterns Self-Analysis Chart 106

SECTION FOUR THE NEW APPROACH **111**

CHAPTER EIGHT: THE HETEROGENEOUS NATURE OF OBESITY ... **113**
 Differences in Unhealthy Attitudes/ Unhealthy Eating Patterns .. 114
 Differences in Motivation 114
 Differences in Expectations 116
 Differences in Patience Level 117

>   *Differences in Resources* *117*
>   *Differences in Biology* *118*
>   *Differences in Confidence* *118*
> **CHAPTER NINE: CHILDHOOD OBESITY** **121**
>   *Stemming the Epidemic* *121*
>   *Basic Principles* *121*
>   *Prevention* *122*
>   *Treatment* *125*
>   *Exercise* *125*
>   *Child Obesity Prevention and Treatment Questionnaire* *126*
>   *Other Directions for the Future* *127*
> **CHAPTER TEN: THE GAME PLAN** **129**
>   *The Content of Our Food* *129*
>   *The Need for Vitamins* *130*
>   *The Role of Bariatric Surgery, Revisited* *131*
>   *The Role of Diets and Weight Loss Programs, Revisited* *132*
>   *Feng's Way, The Game Plan* *133*
>   *Final Thoughts* *138*
> **APPENDIX** **143**
>   *Body Mass Index (BMI) Charts* *143*
> **REFERENCES** **147**
> **GLOSSARY** **157**
> **INDEX** **165**

Preface: Feng's Way to Permanent Weight Loss for Adults and Children

"Discovery consists of seeing what everybody has seen and thinking what nobody has thought." – Albert von Szent-Györgyl (1893-1986)

A Socio-Cultural Approach

This book was begun as an attempt to write a short essay on weight loss for my own patients. With more and more patients wishing to address this issue, I wanted to write something that I would be able to hand to my patients for further contemplation at home when they asked about medically approved ways to lose weight. In all my years as a Medical Doctor I had never felt that any weight loss program or diet made sense. I had always felt that everyone (including the medical community) believed the root cause of weight gain to be caloric imbalance; that it was just a matter of eating more calories than one could use up. There is no question this is <u>how</u> people become overweight but I do not believe it is <u>why</u> people become overweight. I had always felt that there were reasons underlying the caloric imbalance that needed to be addressed as well. As I wrote, my own thoughts started to gel. I had understood almost everything in this book on an intuitive level only but had never organized them and sorted them out in a systematic way. The more I wrote, the more my thoughts gelled until I began to realize that I had enough material for a book. I realized that there was perhaps something of real value here that represented a whole new and different way to approach weight loss.

> Caloric imbalance explains ***how*** people become overweight but not ***why*** they become overweight.

I have come to know a lot of people from all walks of life in my nearly 20 years of experience as a family doctor. I am always telling people that the thing I love most about my job is the fact that very few other jobs allow one to see the full spectrum of humanity. I feel very grateful indeed for the experience. I pride myself as a good listener, and through the years I have learned a lot from my patients. I have come to realize that people become overweight for a great variety of reasons. Because of that, no one method of weight loss will work for everyone. I know that a person who gains a lot of weight after the birth of a child is completely different from someone who has been overweight all her life. A person who eats for emotional reasons and poor self-esteem cannot respond to the same treatment as someone who gained a little excess weight from quitting smoking. The person who overeats for breakfast, lunch and supper is not the same as the person whose extra calories all come from snacks between meals.

I know that people inherit a great deal more from their parents than just genetic material. They also inherit lifestyles, preferences, coping mechanisms and emotional baggage. The prevalence of obesity has been ever on the rise, and I know that there are some very strong cultural and sociological factors at play. It doesn't seem to matter if your heritage is Chinese, Lebanese or Kenyan; when you come to America the incidence of obesity starts to rise. I know that sociological and cultural factors play a very big role in obesity in America.

I use the term obesity often in this book to describe the overweight. It is not my intention to offend by using this word, as almost everything I say regarding the obese also is applicable to the mild to moderately overweight. The official definition of obesity is a BMI (Body Mass Index) of 30 or higher while normal is a BMI of 25 or less, with a BMI of 25 to 30 classified as overweight (for an explanation of BMI's, please see Appendix at the back of the book). For the purposes of this book they can be treated similarly.

This book was written to fill a need that I identified. None of the methods of weight loss that I have come across addresses what I consider to be the root causes of obesity (or the overweight condition if you prefer). Also, few if any of the existing weight loss programs offer any insight on how we might stem the epidemic of obesity and how we might be able to keep our children from becoming overweight. I try to address all of these issues.

I try to show the great variety of reasons for people to be overweight and the rationale for needing different types of treatments. I propose my system of interventions that can be tailored for the different causes of weight problems. I try to instill the notion that if we are to keep our kids from continuing the trend of obesity which we are currently experiencing, we need to recognize that our culturally and sociologically determined attitudes toward food need to change. While I have made every attempt to be as complete as possible, this book makes no claim to be the final word on weight loss. More than anything, this book is meant to start us thinking in a new and different way about our weight problems. These thoughts that I have put down on paper represent my impressions of how obesity works. While some academics may take issue with some of the things I say or with some of my methods, I believe that few will disagree with my basic tenets.

This book was primarily written for the lay person, but an attempt to appeal to academics and health care professionals, including other physicians, was also kept in mind. No book can be all things to all people. I include a glossary at the back of the book to explain some of the medical terms I use. There is also an index to make it easier to find certain parts of the book you may wish to reference or to re-read. For the academically inclined or for those who wish to get more information, I have also included a reference section showing the studies that support some of what I say. I break the references into different topics, allowing for easier verification as well as a short note on some of the studies to show what information I used from the study. Some of the studies appear in more than one section as they were relevant in more than one area.

I considered it to be beyond the scope of this book to be discussing medical diets such as diabetic diets or cholesterol-lowering diets. If your physician has you on one of these diets you obviously need to follow instructions, but you should find that they do not conflict with this book, as this book does not tell you what to eat. It concentrates on why you eat.

The main focus of this book is on health and medical reasons for weight loss rather than on aesthetics. There is nothing wrong with wanting to lose some weight to look better as long as we do it in a manner that is healthy. Weight loss and aesthetics are integrally linked. In fact, I try to show in this book that body image indeed plays a big role in creating expectations and changing the way we think about food as well as the way we eat. Indirectly, I believe this is responsible for a lot of the weight gain problems in our society. However, I mention this here because I also considered it to be beyond the scope of this book to delve into body image issues such as anorexia nervosa or liposuction.

With the ever increasing incidence of obesity, there is a tremendous interest in weight loss. There is hardly a magazine or news tabloid at supermarket checkouts that does not boast some new way to lose weight. Conventional methods of weight loss involving diet and exercise have met with very limited success. These conventional methods have certainly not helped to slow down the epidemic of obesity. This book represents a complete departure from conventional ways we think about weight loss. I believe that we have not been asking the right questions. We have always assumed that the reason some people are overweight is because they eat too much but have not bothered to ask why they eat too much. We have tried to treat the problem of abnormal weight with behaviors that are even more abnormal. It is my belief that this book begins to ask some of the right questions and my hope is that it will start us off in the proper direction to permanent weight loss.

Simon F. Feng, MD
Fall, 2003

SECTION ONE

The Problem

Chapter One: The Goal

"There is nothing that is a more certain sign of insanity than to do the same thing over and over and expect the results to be different" - Einstein

Permanent Weight Loss

As a practicing physician, I am frequently approached by patients wishing to lose weight. They often come in saying things such as, "Doctor, my friend started on this new diet and lost 20 pounds!" or "My sister went on some diet and lost 35 pounds" or "My co-worker started this herbal supplement that is working really well, and he has already lost 25 pounds!" None of these ever impresses me. If, however, a patient were to tell me of someone who lost a significant amount of weight and kept it off for two or three years, I would be all ears. What good is it to lose 20 pounds only to gain back 25? What we should always be striving for is permanent weight loss. On rare occasions I have had patients tell me "All I want is to lose 15 pounds in three months so that I can fit into my wedding dress." However, I think most of us want a permanent result. Even those who claim to want only a temporary weight loss would rather lose the weight permanently if they could.

I tell my patients that we would all love to find a job that we would only have to work at for three or four months (and preferably not have to work very hard at) but get paid for the rest of our lives. That would be awesome, wouldn't it? However, that isn't very likely at all. If we want a paycheck ten years from now, more than likely we will need to be working ten years from now. Weight loss is similar. It would be wonderful to imagine going on some diet that is really easy, sticking to that diet for a couple of months, watching the pounds just melt off and then keeping the weight off for the rest of your life. That would really be nice, wouldn't it? Unfortunately, that is just not very likely. You simply can't expect a permanent result from a temporary change. That's like living in Alaska, taking a vacation to Hawaii in the winter time and expecting warm tropical weather back in Alaska upon your return.

SIMON FENG, M.D.

It follows that if permanent weight loss is what we want, then whatever method of weight loss we employ, the method must still be in effect in ten years if you expect the results to be. If you take an appetite suppressant and lose a bunch of weight, are you prepared to stay on appetite suppressants long term? What happens if you go off them? You find yourself back in Alaska! The same thing applies if you lose weight on a diet - what happens after you reach your "target weight"? If you go off your diet at that time all the weight is coming back! Same result for herbal weight loss.

> You cannot expect a permanent result from a temporary change. If you want to maintain weight loss for 10 years, the method you use must still be in effect in 10 years.

What about bariatric surgery? In brief, bariatric surgery is surgery to rearrange the anatomy of your digestive tract to induce weight loss. It will be discussed in a later chapter. Well, if you have your stomach by-passed, ten years from now your stomach will still be by-passed. Therefore, this method at least can be a permanent method of weight loss (which the research shows). It is, however, quite a drastic step with very significant possible complications and risks. Nevertheless, I believe that it is justified for some patients. We'll get back to this in a later chapter.

Can you continue appetite suppressants long term? That is probably not such a good idea, and most of the time even if you continue on the medications long-term, the weight tends to start gradually coming back after about six months. Appetite suppressants also tend to increase your blood pressure and heart rate, which increase your cardiovascular disease risks, especially long-term. Herbal appetite suppressants and metabolism boosters are equally unsafe if not more so. There is also the high financial cost of taking medication long-term.

Many patients tell me they just want me to give them medications to give them a head-start, then they promise to eat better after that to maintain their weight loss. The problem with that is: **if they don't have the initiative and incentive to eat properly when they are overweight, where is their initiative and incentive to eat properly going to come from when they have already lost the weight that they want to lose**? It doesn't get any easier to eat properly after the weight is lost. They may think that losing weight is harder than keeping the weight off, but in reality it is much easier to lose the weight than to keep it off. Think of all the yo-yo diets people go on.

> One may think that losing weight is harder than keeping the weight off, but in reality, it is much easier to lose the weight than to keep it off.

Ideally, we would really like to find a permanent method of weight loss that does not require surgery or long-term medications. It would be an added bonus if we could maintain our weight loss without a struggle and would not have to be battling weight gain for the rest of our lives. I believe this may be possible with my approach.

The Law of Conservation of Energy

The Law of Conservation of Energy is one of the very basic physical laws that explain the physical world we live in. It basically states that energy can be converted from one form to another but is never created or lost. We can turn electrical energy into light or heat, we can change sunlight into heat or electricity or we can release stored chemical energy into heat. However, we can never create new energy or destroy existing energy.

Weight loss is always a function of energy balance. You have energy coming in as calories and energy going out as calories. It's like your bank account: if more money comes into your account than goes out, your balance should be getting fatter. If it doesn't, someone is stealing money from you. On the other hand, if more money goes out of your account than comes in, your account balance has to be shrinking, unless you have an illegal source of income the IRS does not know about. Similarly, if you take in more energy in the way of calories than you use up, your energy account balance (i.e. your weight) goes up. If you spend more calories than you consume, your energy account balance goes down. Simple. This is true even for those patients who truly do have an abnormal metabolism, such as with hypothyroidism. These patients just burn up calories at a slower rate and therefore need fewer calories. In my bank account analogy, these patients are like real tightwads. They never spend more money than the bare minimum. Therefore, it is much easier for their account to grow. However, the Law of Conservation of Energy still holds true. This Law of Conservation of Energy is a physical law that is as hard to violate as the Law of Gravity. I occasionally have patients who try to tell me that they can get fat drinking water, but I have yet to meet the patient who will tell me that the Law of Gravity does not apply to them. These patients may not be aware of where or how their extra calories are coming in; they may not even be aware that these caloreis are coming in at all, but they <u>are</u> coming in.

We also see skinny teenagers who seem to be eating non-stop without getting fat. The important thing to understand here is that they are gaining weight but getting taller as well. Adults who are not getting taller cannot eat like these teenagers without getting fat unless they have an extraordinarily active lifestyle. Invariably, people also tell me of some adult they know who is thin but seems to be able to eat a phenomenal amount of food. The thing to understand here is that while they are able to eat a tremendous amount of food, they do not eat that way all the time. Over the course of one to two weeks they don't eat more than their bodies need to maintain their weights.

I should point out at this time that I am using weight gain as a synonym for fat gain. It is possible for patients to gain weight drinking only water and salt, by retaining water in their systems. This is not fat gain but merely fluid gain. Our weight reflects the weights of our bony skeleton, our organs, our muscles, our blood and other fluids, and of course our fatty tissues. Normally, the weights of our skeleton, muscles, organs, etc. do not change on a day-to-day basis. Hence, if our weight goes up or down by five pounds we can usually assume that we have gained or lost five pounds of fat. This is not always true. Our fluid status can also change very quickly. Our muscle mass may also change fairly quickly. If someone gets into a good exercise program as part of a weight loss program, he or she may lose five pounds of fat but also gain five pounds of muscle with a net weight loss of zero. He or she may feel very disheartened that all that hard work has not resulted in even one pound of weight loss. Fluid gain is also generally considered undesirable but tends to be short term only. You can lose weight by taking a diuretic and making yourself dehydrated, but you will not have lost a single ounce of fat! Not at all what you really want. Anyhow, for the purposes of this book, I really wish to concentrate on fat gain and fat loss, which I will equate with weight gain or weight loss, realizing that the terms are not exactly interchangeable.

From the concept of the Law of Conservation of Energy it follows that weight loss is always possible even if not always easy. I do encounter patients who tell me they gain weight even though they "honestly don't eat enough to keep a bird alive". I believe that many of these patients truly believe that, but what they really have is one or more of the group of unhealthy eating patterns that I shall describe later in this book. What I do know is that if these patients undergo bariatric surgery and have their stomachs by-passed, lo and behold, they start to lose weight! Anytime people are forced to go without sufficient food, whether in a concentration camp or if shipwrecked, they lose weight. It is true that some people gain weight easier than others do, but it is simply not possible to get fat on a negative calorie balance.

In all fairness, there is a subset of patients for whom weight gain is a lot harder to avoid. Any woman who has ever been pregnant will tell you that her appetite goes up. There are medications such as prednisone, as well as some anti-depressants and anti-psychotics, that may in some people cause very significant weight gain. However, even for these cases, the Law of Conservation of Energy still applies.

At this point, it may be appropriate to discuss low-carbohydrate diets, which have become very popular recently. The theory behind these diets is that a low-carbohydrate diet results in a higher metabolism and more efficient use of calories, thereby allowing you to lose weight despite relatively high calorie consumption. This is a very interesting concept but may not be true. A recent extensive review of the literature (involving 3268 participants in 107 studies) showed that low-carbohydrate diets may have been more successful than high-carbohydrate diets because the diets were easier to follow and patients were likely to stay on the diets longer. The reduced carbohydrate intake also resulted *unconsciously* in a lower caloric intake, which was responsible for the weight loss. A pound of cotton wool weighs as much as a pound of nails, and, unfortunately, a calorie from protein can cause the same weight gain as a calorie from carbohydrates.

SIMON FENG, M.D.

I do believe that a diet high in carbohydrates (therefore high in calories) is much more likely to lead to weight gain. I have known quite a few patients as well as personal friends who have lost significant weight following low-carbohydrate diets In a nutshell, these diets allow you to eat meat and vegetables but the carbohydrate intake is severely limited. The main problem with these diets is that most people do not stay on them, even though in the later stages you may be allowed to eat a little carbohydrate. I once saw a survey that asked, "If there was only one food you could eat for the rest of your life what would you choose this food to be?" The answer was not steak or chocolate, or even ice cream, but overwhelmingly, bread. Most people are simply not willing to give up on bread permanently. Also, I do not think of low-carbohydrate diets as "normal" diets because all over the world, the staple food in any culture is some form of carbohydrate. In some cultures it is bread, in others it may be rice or potatoes. Yet, in those cultures obesity is not a problem. For carbohydrates to be such a universally important part of the diet tells me that it is very important, and I suspect that we cannot eliminate it completely with impunity. It also concerns me somewhat that these diets often do not allow fruits.

There is no question that the carbohydrate content in the typical North American diet has increased dramatically over the past several decades. I do think that this excess carbohydrate intake plays a big role in weight gain and the current epidemic of obesity. I agree that excess carbohydrates are not healthy and also not conducive to weight loss. However, I am not sure that eliminating carbohydrates from the diet is the long-term answer to weight problems.

A low-carbohydrate diet in itself is fairly safe. While a small minority of people may be more likely to get kidney stones and the high protein load is probably not great for those with kidney or liver disease, most people tolerate it well. If you feel that you can stick to this kind diet forever, go ahead. As I will demonstrate later in the book, I believe that people are different and become overweight for different reasons. Hence, different treatments work for different people. If a low-carbohydrate diet is working for you on a long-term basis, there is probably no reason to stop doing it. As the adage goes, "Never argue with success." My solution, on the other hand, seeks to identify the root cause of the overweight condition and tries to normalize the eating pattern so that we can enjoy foods from <u>all</u> of the food groups.

The Problem with Diets

We often hear people say things like, "This diet really works!" or, "I have never found a diet that worked for me." What do they mean? When do we say a diet works? If someone loses 20 pounds on a diet, did it work? If that person gains back all 20 pounds in the next 6 months, did the diet work?

Because I define success as permanent weight loss, I do not consider any diet a success if the weight does not stay off. For example, if a diet allowed you to eat all the grapefruit you wanted (or could stand) but didn't allow any other kind of food, you would lose a lot of weight very fast, but it is not a diet that you could stay on very long. You could say that the diet "worked" because it made you lose weight, or that it "didn't work" because the weight did not stay off. I guess that what I am trying to say is that diets can make you lose weight but cannot make you keep the weight off.

> Diets can help you lose weight but cannot make you keep the weight off.

Can diets ever work long term? Yes, but only when they are viewed as a permanent change or what I call a "Dietary Way of Life". I have had patients who completely changed their lives around following a heart attack or similar catastrophe. These people made some serious changes in their life. Often they are people who have smoked for 30 years or more and have failed repeated attempts to quit smoking but finally quit after they suffered a heart attack. They start eating the way they should and start exercising regularly. This time they succeed in losing weight and keeping it off because they finally realize that this is the way they are going to be eating for the rest of their lives. They have changed their diet into a "Dietary Way of Life".

If you are one of the few who have successfully lost weight through dieting and managed to keep it off for many years, please continue to do so. I am not saying that it is impossible to lose weight by dieting but just that it is very difficult indeed.

Another problem with dieting is actually malnutrition. This is especially true for "yo-yo" dieters. When they are on a crash diet, they are not getting enough minerals such as calcium or iron, vitamins or essential amino acids. Once they go off their diets, they often gain their weight back eating junk foods such as candy bars, ice cream or other sweets. Again, these foods have little nutritive value. They don't get their vitamins losing weight and they don't get them gaining weight back. If this goes on for some time, they become malnourished even though they are overweight!

The biggest problem with diets, however, is what I call the diet mentality, which I believe causes more problems. This will be discussed later in Chapter Six.

How about Exercise?

Exercise is essential and should be a part of any weight loss program whenever possible. Studies show time and again that almost always, the people who have a regular exercise program are far more likely to succeed in losing weight on a long-term basis.

However, exercise by itself does not work unless it is coupled to proper eating. The reason for this is that our bodies are too efficient. It is disheartening to realize that you can run one mile and put back all the calories with just one glass of milk. Exercise is important, but you cannot simply exercise your way to weight loss without modifying how you eat. There is evidence that the amount of exercise needed to make a significant impact on your weight is about 60 minutes per day of moderate activity, which is like running 4 to 5 miles everyday!

I do not want to be misunderstood here. I strongly endorse exercise in any weight loss program. However, there are people who have a real aversion toward exercise or cannot exercise for one reason or another (for example, severe arthritis). If they feel that they *have* to exercise in order to succeed in weight loss, they will feel that it is impossible for them. I do not wish these people to feel disenfranchised, but at the same time I do not wish to give anyone the idea that they do not need to exercise.

The other thing I would like to say about a regular exercise program is that a formal program is much better than a home program. America has too many basements with exercise equipment gathering dust. The reason for this is not usually because the equipment is ineffective. When you have insomnia and find yourself watching an infomercial on TV at 3:00 a.m. touting a piece of exercise equipment, they will often tell you how their equipment compares favorably, or perhaps is identical to those found in high-priced health clubs costing $500 - $1,000 a year to belong to. What they tell you is usually true. The problem is actually this: if you pay $500 a year to belong to a club, you promise yourself to go after work Mondays, Wednesdays and Fridays, and by golly you show up! When the equipment is at home in your basement, you may fully intend to use it. Unfortunately, just when you are about to, you realize that, "I almost forgot! Oprah comes on in 5 minutes!" and you decide you'll exercise after that program. You know what I mean. It is precisely because of convenience that you want home exercise equipment, and the reason that you won't use it is precisely because it is too convenient. It is just too easy to postpone it for an hour, or a day. After a while the equipment just gets forgotten. The only sure way to use home equipment is to schedule the exercise into your day very firmly and stick to it. You must schedule the exact time and the duration of your exercise program, perhaps scheduled around your favorite show which you can watch from your treadmill. You must schedule your dinners, movies and parties around it, making exceptions only when absolutely necessary and reschedule any exercise routine you missed for another time. Better still, make the commitment to wake up 30 minutes earlier and make exercise a fixed part of your daily morning routine.

Cures vs. Controls

In my medical practice I am always trying to differentiate for my patients the difference between cures and controls. If you have appendicitis and the surgeon removes the appendix, it is cured. If you have pneumonia and we clear it up with antibiotics, it is cured. If you go on birth control pills to prevent unwanted pregnancies, we are controlling your fertility but certainly not curing it. If you shave your facial hair every day and you haven't had a beard in ten years, can

SIMON FENG, M.D.

you stop shaving? Have you cured your beard growth? Of course not.

If you need to take medicines for diabetes or high cholesterol, can you ever stop the medicines? Well, actually that depends. I tell my patients if they succeed in making a significant and permanent lifestyle change, then it is possible that they may not require the medications anymore. For example, I have had patients who lost over 100 pounds after bariatric surgery and didn't require their medications any longer. In fact, many of them did not require medications immediately following surgery because the way they ate had changed drastically immediately after surgery. Another patient became a vegetarian and was able to get off all her medications. One other patient I remember retired from interstate truck driving, where it was very difficult to eat properly. He started a regular exercise program and began eating healthier and no longer had the same high caffeine intake of his truck-driving days. Not surprisingly, he also no longer needed his high blood pressure pills. I also remember patients who recovered from alcoholism or drug abuse or quit smoking and were able to reduce or eliminate their medicines. In all these cases they "cured" their high blood pressure by making some life-altering changes. On the other hand, if you are going to eat the same way, live the same lifestyle and change nothing, why do you think that you will not need your medications in ten years? To paraphrase Einstein, insanity is doing exactly the same thing over and over again and expecting a different result next time. (A note of caution for the readers: *do not stop any of your medications without consulting your doctor or health care provider.* Even if you have completely changed the way you eat and have already lost 50 pounds, you still need to make sure that you are monitored closely when going off medications.)

When planning your weight loss, ask yourself if you are going for a cure or if you are trying to control it. If you are going to only control your weight, you face a life-long battle with it and you must never get off your program. It becomes like shaving; keep shaving as long as you do not want the hair growth. On the other hand, if you want to "cure" your weight problem, we need to find the cause of the problem and see if we can't fix it.

My slogan is "If you want to lose weight permanently you have to learn to act and think like a normal weight person, *not* like a fat person trying to lose weight!" People without weight problems do not go on diets, do not count calories and most certainly do not take any appetite-suppressants. The only people doing these things are people with weight problems. Why should we be emulating people with weight problems instead of people without weight problems? This book was the product of trying to find the underlying causes of obesity to see if it can't be corrected. I am of the firm belief that for almost everyone, if they could only learn to eat like a normal weight person, they would eventually normalize their weight. Why can't we eat like that normal weight person, or can we? Is there some abnormality in how we eat and can we cure it?

> If you want to lose weight permanently you have to learn to act and think like a normal weight person, *not* like a fat person trying to lose weight.

For every overweight person that you find for me, I will be able to find someone the same race, same age, same sex, same height, same number of children, and same occupation but not overweight. Why is there this difference between these two people? From my discussion above on the Law of Conservation of Energy, we know that the overweight one eats more than the other one, but my question is more basic than that. The person without the weight problem also enjoys good food. He or she also eats pizzas and hamburgers, chocolates and ice cream, yet does not have a weight problem. People without weight problems enjoy their food every bit as much as their overweight counterparts, and probably even more so because they can enjoy their food without any sense of guilt or shame. We know that overweight people eat too much, but my question is why? What causes them to over-consume? If we do not understand the reasons for the over-consumption but merely tell them to eat less, how can we succeed?

> For every overweight person that you find for me, I will be able to find someone the same race same age, same sex, same height, same number of children, and same occupation but not overweight. Why is there this difference between the two people?

This book is an attempt to answer that question. When my friends found out that I was writing a book on weight loss, many of them wanted to know what my "secret" to weight loss was. I believe that the answer to permanent weight loss is not to be found in *what* we eat but in *why* we eat. Overweight people over-consume because they eat for the wrong reasons. If we can get them to stop eating for the wrong reasons and start eating for the right reasons they will lose weight permanently. They will be able to do so without making many sacrifices.

Overview of the Book

Section One of this book (The Problem), comprises the first two chapters. In this chapter, I defined the challenge we face as that of finding a weight loss solution that will yield *permanent* results. Chapter Two, discussing the current epidemic of obesity, plays a major role in the formation of my ideas.

Section Two of the book (Current Treatments and Philosophies) deals with the current philosophies and strategies of weight loss, as well as some of the reasons why they have not proven to be as successful as one would like. Chapter Four discusses the currently available approaches to weight loss, as well as their shortcomings, and is essential to understanding the rest of my book.

Section Three of the book (A New Viewpoint) presents my ideas as to what I consider to be the real causes of obesity. I show how unhealthy attitudes and unhealthy eating patterns are the real culprits that explain the epidemic of obesity.

Section Four (The New Approach) offers my suggestions for treating the newly recognized disorders. This Section also presents my solutions for addressing childhood obesity and its epidemic, which are areas that sadly lack any good treatment options today.

As you read this book, you will find that certain key ideas get repeated, sometimes more than once, in different chapters of the book. One reason for this is that I anticipate people may wish to re-read certain chapters and not others. The book will not always be read from beginning to end in order, even though I have tried to organize the book in a logical flow.

Chapter Two: The Epidemic of Obesity

"We each day dig our graves with our teeth." – Samuel Smiles 1812-1904

The Scope of the Problem

Many of us have heard of the epidemic of obesity. I was aware of the statistics, but when I saw the maps charting this epidemic, I was still shocked. On the next few pages are six maps showing how obesity has increased over the 15 short years from 1986 to 2001. The maps plot out the prevalence of obesity (how common obesity is among in the general public), with obesity being defined as someone having a Body Mass Index (BMI) of 30 or higher, which is roughly equivalent to a 5'4" person being 30 pounds overweight. (BMI is a measure of weight and height that gives us a measure of how fat a person is. Please see Appendix for more information on BMI.) Each map is three years from the last. It is a truly shocking demonstration of the epidemic of obesity to see visually the march of obesity across the face of the nation. When you realize that nine states have moved from the category of less than 10% obesity in 1986, to 20-25% *in a mere 15 years,* it is downright scary. In 1986, no state had more than 15% obesity but today, not a single state has less than 15% obesity! By 2001, one out of four people in Mississippi was obese! Where will we be in another 15 years?

How bad is this? After all, nobody dies of obesity, do they? Well, not directly, in the sense that very few people have "terminal obesity" listed on their death certificate. However, obesity is very closely related to diabetes, high blood pressure and heart disease, and people *do* die of those diseases. When you consider how closely obesity is tied to these diseases, you can begin to appreciate the impact this epidemic is going to have on us over the next decade or so.

These other diseases often take many years after developing before they start causing problems such as heart attacks and strokes. In other words, after a person develops high blood pressure, it may take up to 20 years before the high blood pressure has done

SIMON FENG, M.D.

enough damage to cause a heart attack or stroke. People who became obese in the mid-1980's or early 1990's may only now be starting to get heart attacks today. The people just becoming obese today will be showing up in the emergency rooms over the next 10 to 15 years with their heart attacks. What we see now as the epidemic of obesity is only the very tip of the iceberg. Before very long, it will turn into an epidemic of heart attacks and strokes. It is just the first wave of a hurricane to come.

Little has been done to stem this future wave of health problems. There is not even a defined plan to deal with this epidemic. If this were any other disease, the public outcry would be deafening. Imagine if the maps revealed the spread of West Nile Virus or SARS. While obesity does not have the short-term mortality rate of SARS, it plays a huge role in the top killers in America, namely heart attacks, diabetes, strokes. The impact of obesity on the health of the nation is immeasurably higher than that of West Nile Virus. The cost of health care attributable to obesity is possibly higher than that of smoking.

FENG'S WAY: TO PERMANENT WEIGHT LOSS

Prevalence of Obesity (Maps)

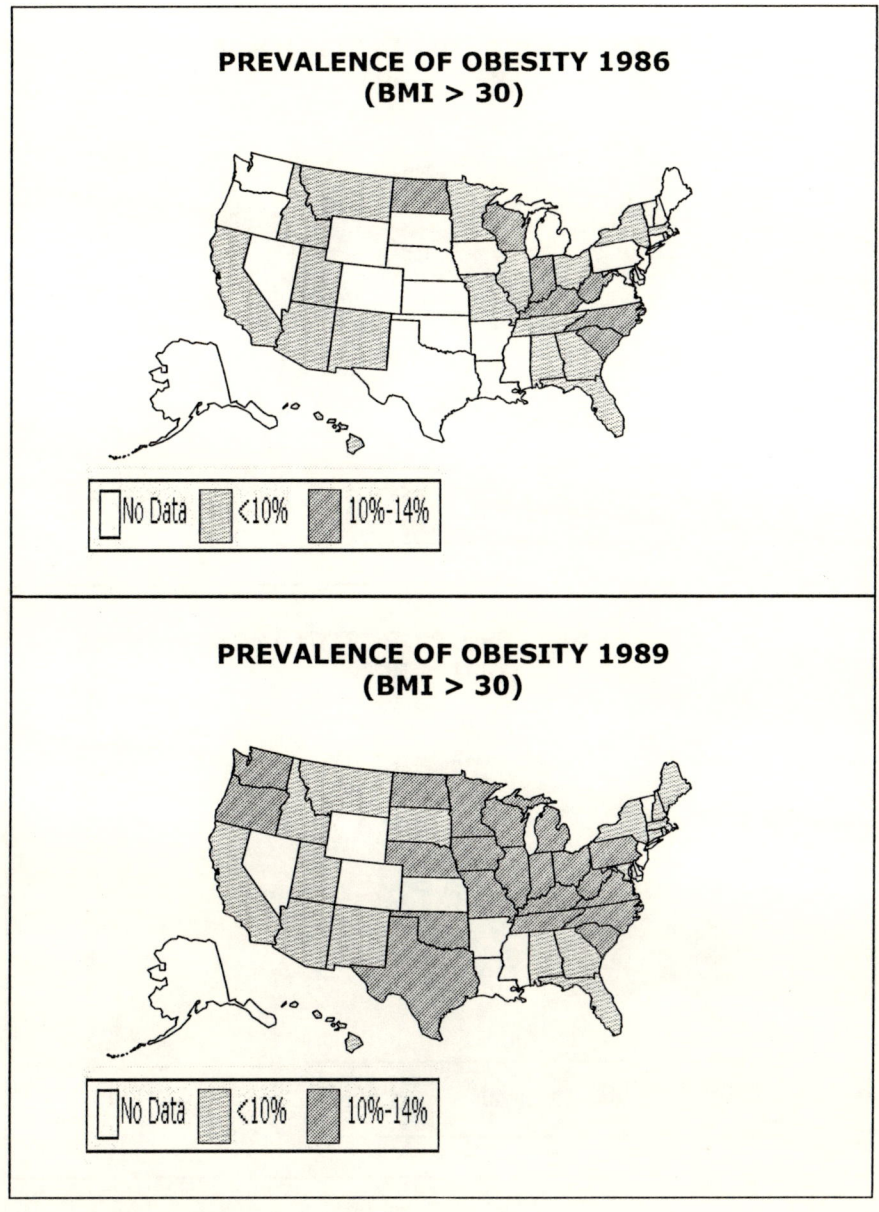

SIMON FENG, M.D.

Prevalence of Obesity (Maps)

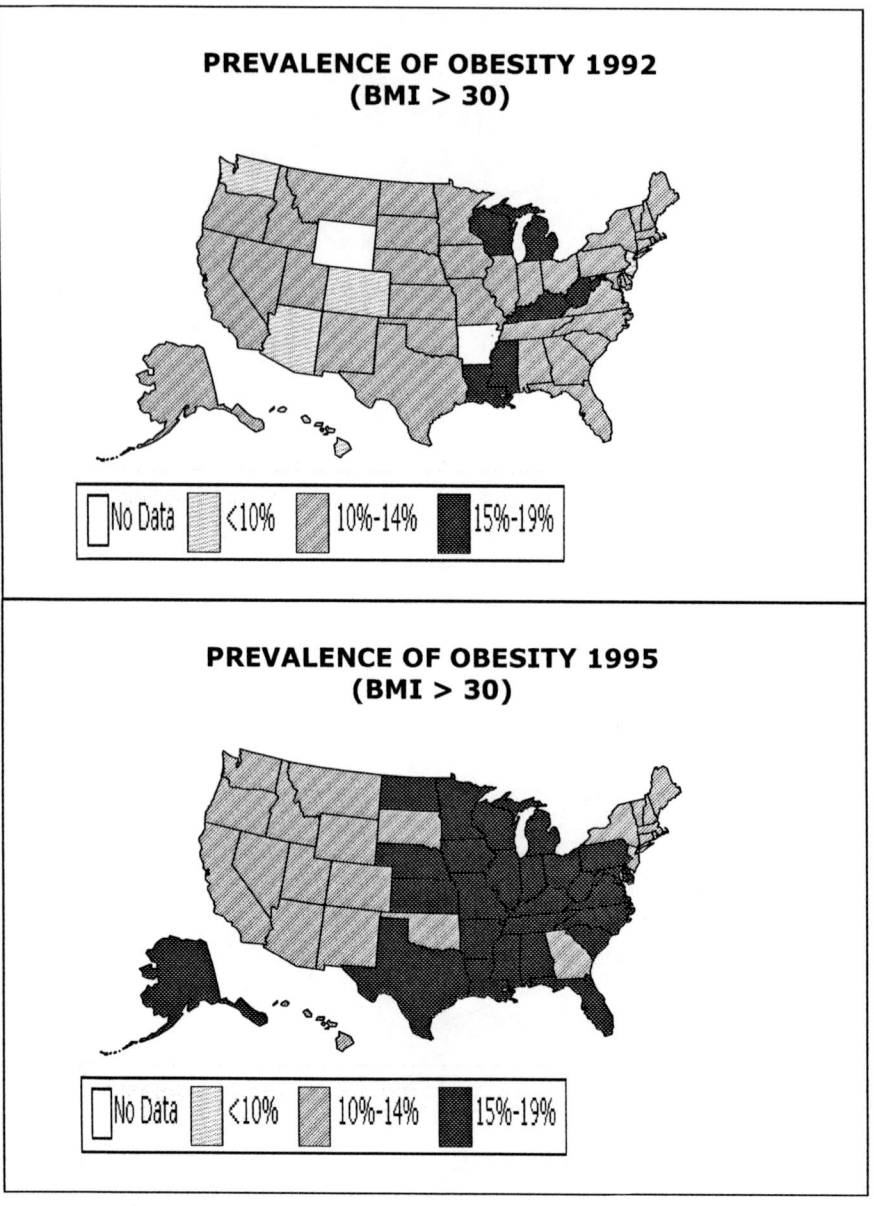

FENG'S WAY: TO PERMANENT WEIGHT LOSS

Prevalence of Obesity (Maps)

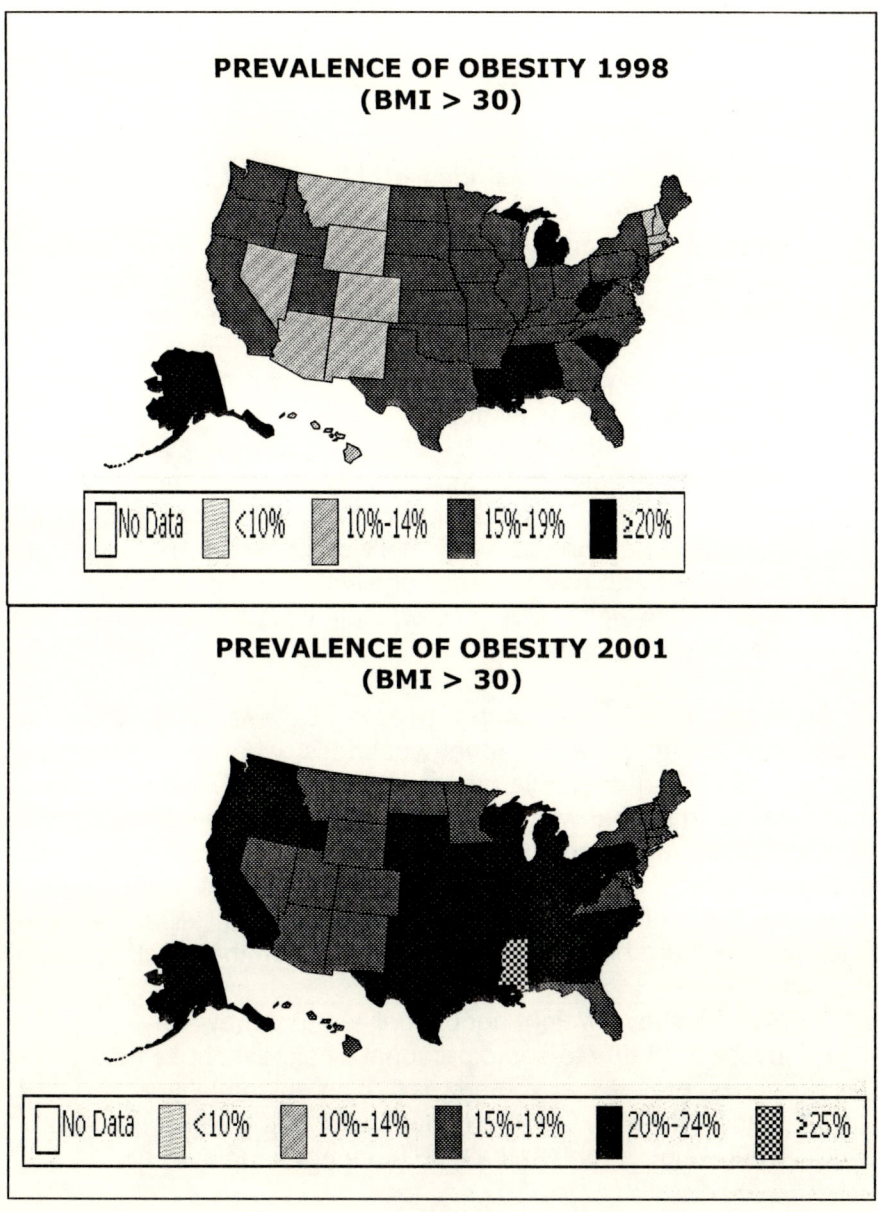

Source: Mokdad AH et al, JAMA 1999; 282:16, JAMA 2001; 286:10, JAMA 2003; 289:1

Why this Epidemic is Silent

Why has the epidemic of obesity been relatively silent and why has there been no public outcry? I believe that it is because of several factors:

1. The public has no real idea of the severity of the epidemic, nor of the significance of it.
2. Obesity is uncomfortable to think about and often politically incorrect to talk about.
3. The disease takes a long time to kill the patient and because of that, there is no public panic.
4. It is not a contagious disease so it does not fit our notions of what an epidemic is all about.
5. The cause of obesity is perceived by most people to be either genetic/metabolic (bad luck if you inherited this from your parents but unaffected people do not have to worry) or due to poor lifestyle choices (and therefore deserved). Again, not consistent with how we traditionally think of epidemics.
6. Most overweight people view their weight problem as their private personal demon.

Although most overweight people believe that they are overweight due to some personal weakness, when you realize that you are part of an epidemic, you should realize that there may be factors involved in your weight problem that you have not been aware of. Could these factors be the reasons that you have not been able to lose weight? One person could become obese from personal weakness but is the whole nation becoming weak all at the same time? Surely there has to be a better explanation than that.

> Most overweight people believe that they are overweight due to some personal weakness, but when you realize that you are part of an epidemic, you should realize that there may be factors involved in your weight problem that you have not been aware of.

I also do not believe that the cause of this epidemic of obesity is genetic or metabolic. This is not to say that nobody is overweight because of genetic or metabolic disorders, but it is obvious from the rapid pace of this epidemic that it cannot possibly be explained by genetic or metabolic problems alone. There is no way a genetic condition can be turned into an epidemic. It is just not possible. Can you imagine an epidemic of blue eyes?

Consider also that the above maps span only 15 years – less than one generation! How could genetics explain this when, for the most part, we are talking about the same people with the same genes that they had 15 years ago?

Those of you who are not overweight, consider this: If it's not genetics and it is not just personal weakness, how safe are you really from this epidemic? How safe are your children?

If it is not genetics and not just personal weakness, what else is there? If we can identify this other factor (or factors) in the epidemic of obesity, can we use it to help us lose weight and stop this epidemic?

I believe that I understand what these factors are, and this knowledge can help us lose weight. Yes, it may even possibly help stop the epidemic.

What Can Be Done?

The first principle of dealing with any epidemic is "containment". We must find a way to protect the unaffected. In other words, we must start with prevention. In order to do this, we must understand how this disease spreads. At the risk of seeming immodest, I believe that I understand the true reasons behind this epidemic, and this understanding can help direct us toward both prevention and treatment. It is my wish to not only help people with their personal weight problems but also to begin to tackle the problem of the epidemic.

There are many weight loss programs out there trying to help overweight people lose weight. I would like to point out that the epidemic of obesity has marched along despite all the diet and exercise books ever written, as well as all the weight loss clinics in existence. In my opinion, we will never make a dent in the epidemic

SIMON FENG, M.D.

of obesity if we concentrate only on the treatment and not on the prevention as well. As you read this book, you may come to realize that it has also been written with normal weight people in mind, so that they may understand why people become overweight. I discuss childhood obesity and the sociology of obesity as I believe that these also hold the key to success in fighting this epidemic. By understanding why people become overweight we can hopefully prevent our children from becoming overweight, and just by doing this, we can wipe out this epidemic in one generation.

> In my opinion, we will never make a dent in the epidemic of obesity if we concentrate only on the treatment and not on the prevention as well.

The good news is that the same understanding of why people gain weight also gives us the key to treating personal weight problems. We will get to that in Section Three (Chapter Six).

SECTION TWO

Current Treatment Philosophies

Chapter Three: Herbal Weight Loss and Natural Dietary Supplements

"I will use treatment to help the sick according to my ability and judgment, but I will never use treatment to injure or wrong them" – part of the Hippocratic Oath taken by many physicians.

Popularity of Herbal/Nutritional Supplements

There is no scarcity of "natural" products out there that purport to help you lose weight. By claiming to be herbal they do not fall under the jurisdiction of the Food and Drug Administration (FDA). There is something very disarming and somehow very seductive about being a natural herbal product. It implies implicitly if not explicitly that these products are safe and less toxic, with less or no drug interactions, environmentally friendly, and intrinsically good and not evil. After all, how could Mother Nature ever hurt you, unlike evil, toxic technology?

As an added bonus, these products can be bought without a prescription so that you could buy it in secret without any embarrassment. Nobody needs to know that you are trying to lose weight; if you fail no one will think less of you. You do not need to announce to anyone "I am obese and I need help", in the same way that alcoholics have to announce their alcoholism at AA meetings.

These herbal remedies have become mainstream in several ways. They are now advertised on prime time television and radio, which gives these products a veneer of respectability they didn't have when the products were advertised only in the back of magazines. The nutritional supplement industry hires well-known people such as syndicated talk show hosts to endorse their products. The public seems to believe that if it is on prime time it must be legitimate. Surely it can't be false if it is on national TV! They imagine that there must be some sort of governmental agency looking after their interests. Well, there is no such agency. Nutritional supplements and herbs are not regulated by the Food and Drug Administration.

SIMON FENG, M.D.

Myths and Misconceptions about Herbal Remedies in General

First, I would like to point out that I really do not wish to come across as being anti-herbal. Being of Chinese heritage, I grew up with herbal medications at home. I remember growing up with the smells of the brewing of various herbal concoctions. I do know that some herbal medications can work - I do not dispute that. What I have a problem with is what I consider to be unsubstantiated claims associated with herbal remedies. I would like to dispel some common myths about herbal medications. As you read this, I trust that you will understand that it is not really herbal remedies that I am complaining about, but rather the unscrupulous conduct of many herbal remedy companies and the way they exploit the public because of these frequently held myths. This section is not just about herbal weight loss but also about herbal/dietary supplements in general. Almost everything that I say about herbal remedies also applies to nutritional supplements.

Myth #1. Herbal medicines are safer than conventional medications.

There is often a feeling that if it is natural, it can't hurt you. In fact, I have often heard such claims made of herbal remedies. As it turns out, the most potent toxins known to man are all natural. Botulism toxin is completely natural but one of the most potent toxins known to man. The second most potent toxin known to man is tetanus toxin, also 100% natural. South American Indians used to tip their arrows with tubocurare, which is so toxic that a light coating on the tip of an arrow is enough to kill a man. If you pick the wrong kind of mushrooms you can get very sick or even die if you get enough of it. If natural plants are harmless, would you like a tossed salad of poison ivy?

> Many of the most potent toxins known to man are natural.

I like to point out that cocaine is a natural product but can easily kill in an overdose. Tobacco is of course also an herbal product, isn't it? I know you don't smoke most herbal products, but remember that chewing tobacco can cause mouth cancers, digestive cancers and bladder cancers. How many other herbals can cause cancers that we do not know about?

> Tobacco is also an herbal product but can cause various cancers. How many other herbals can cause cancers that we do not know about?

What about allergies? Most people are unaware that the Echinacea they take for a cold is cross-allergenic with ragweed. This means that if they were actually suffering from ragweed allergies instead of the cold, they could be making themselves worse rather than better. If they are allergic to Echinacea they may also be allergic to Feverfew (which is used to treat migraine headaches and also, ironically, used to treat allergies). Patients are unlikely to be aware of these cross-allergenic ties, as they probably will not be consulting any professional such as an herbalist or pharmacist. People die from peanut allergies; could the same fate befall patients with allergies to herbal medications?

I also like to point out that many conventional medicines started out as herbal medicines. We derived aspirin from willow bark, digitalis from foxglove and atropine from belladonna. Yet all these medications have definite side effects and toxicity.

I tell my patients that there is no magic in herbs. If St. John's wort does something for you that spinach does not, it is because St. John's wort contains a chemical that you don't find in spinach. Exactly like any other biologically-active chemical (whether we are talking about alcohol or marijuana or caffeine), you need a certain level for it to have the desired effect but too much could run you into toxicity. I have seen products that I consider to be ridiculous, such as St. John's wort lipstick or St. John's wort potato chips. How many of those potato chips are you supposed to take? Do you get into toxic levels if you eat the whole bag?

There is really no question that herbal medications can hurt you or even kill you. The best known of these is ephedra or ma-huang. This is of course the active herbal ingredient of many or most herbal weight loss preparations. It suppresses the appetite while it cranks up the body's metabolism and "burns up fat". The FDA believes ephedra has killed many athletes, including Baltimore Orioles pitching prospect, Steve Bechler.

SIMON FENG, M.D.

> There is really no question that herbal medications can hurt you or even kill you.

As another example, herbal products that claim to increase breast size may contain compounds called phytoestrogens or plant-derived estrogens. No physician would advocate that you rub estrogen cream on your breasts or take estrogen pills to increase breast size because of the known link between estrogens and breast cancer as well as uterine cancer. We really do not have sufficient evidence that phytoestrogens are any safer. I would strongly suspect that if the compounds truly do have enough activity in the breast to increase breast size, they would have to increase your chances of breast cancer.

Myth #2. Herbal medicines are natural

Thirty years ago, if you wanted an herbal remedy, it was probably collected from where the plant grew naturally. That is now no longer the case. Herbal medicine plants are now grown as commercial plants, and are traded as a commodity, just like coffee or beans. They are grown on farms where they are sprayed with pesticides, herbicides, insecticides and fertilizers. After the crop is harvested there is probably only a minimal degree of processing, if any, to remove residues of chemical pesticides or herbicides. Consider this: it is recommended that you wash your fruits and vegetables before consumption. It is very possible that residual quantities of these chemicals can be found in commercially-grown herbal medicines. Occasional use of these products may not be of any significance but I cannot believe chronic ingestion can be good for you.

> Herbal medicine plants are now grown as commercial plants on farms where they are sprayed with pesticides, herbicides, insecticides and fertilizers.

Many herbal preparations also contain preservatives and stabilizers. Because the products are biological, there is usually the problem of the product spoiling. These additives can also be a source of allergic reactions. In higher amounts they may cause other health problems and may even prove to be carcinogenic. On the other hand, if the herbal product does not have any preservatives, you must be concerned about spoilage.

Myth #3. Herbal medicines are standardized.

Plants such as St. John's wort, ginseng or gingko are now grown all over the world, from the orient to South America to Canada and Europe. No one really knows whether gingko from Canada really does the same thing as gingko from South America or New Zealand.

We know that plant characteristics are very much dependent on the environment they grow in. For example, it is well known that coffee beans in Columbia grown in the mountains produce much better flavor than coffee beans grown at sea level in the same country. The same strain of maple tree produces superior maple syrup in Vermont than it would in Washington State. Can we assume that the same herb from Canada has the same activity as one from the Ukraine?

Does it matter if you harvest gingko leaves in the spring or in the fall? The leaves don't even look the same. They are green in the spring and yellow in the fall, so I can't quite imagine that they will have the same medicinal value. How much of the stalk must be taken? Does it matter if you use freeze-dried leaves?

To make things much more complicated, botanicals often come in different strains. Think about apples. There are so many varieties from Gala to Granny Smiths. Some apples are suitable only for cooking. How many different strains of Saw Palmetto are there? Do they all work the same? Is two grams of the whole berry of one strain of Saw Palmetto the same as two grams of a different strain? Even if they get a "standardized" lipophilic extract, does it matter where the berries were grown?

Botanicals often come in different strains. Do they all work the same?

It was reported in the November 1995 issue of <u>Consumer Reports</u> that two different brands of ginseng, both labeled as having 648 mg of ginseng, when tested in the laboratory showed that one brand

SIMON FENG, M.D.

actually had ten times more active ingredient, ginsenoside, than the other brand.

Further complicating matters, remember how I told you that herbals are traded like a commodity? Well, most herbal companies do not own their own farms but buy their plants on the open market. This means that if they can get a cheaper price from New Zealand this year, but previous plants came from South America, the same brand may now be radically different. Different lot numbers of the same brand with the same packaging can still be completely different in activity.

I don't really see the solution to this unless herbal companies are required to purify the active chemical ingredient and sell their products by the amount of active ingredient. However, it is extremely unlikely that this will happen and if it did, it would seem too much like conventional medications.

Myth #4. Herbal medications have little or no side effects

The previous section discussed how herbal medications work due to the fact that they contain a certain biologically-active chemical. From that, it should become obvious that side effects are also unavoidable. Even regular foods can have side effects. For example, we know that coffee can give you insomnia, spicy foods can give you heartburn, beets can give your urine a red tint, licorice can have a diuretic effect, and many others. I do not understand how some people can claim that natural products are completely free of side-effects. What is true is that most herbal preparations are not purified and therefore usually not very potent. This lack of potency means that it is usually associated with only mild to moderate side effects, but it also means that it is usually useful only for treating mild to moderate symptoms. If you made the herbal preparation more concentrated and more potent you will also see an increase in the severity of side effects.

Many people are very concerned about the long list of side effects printed on the sheet from the pharmacy when they get a conventional medicine. The FDA requires these side effects to be reported. I was an investigator in a study several years ago involving a new antibiotic being submitted for FDA approval. The experience with the FDA was quite enlightening. As investigators, we were instructed to report any adverse event, *whether or not we thought the event was due to the medication.* Our instructions stated specifically that *causality was not to be considered* in deciding to report the event. We had a patient in the study who took only one dose of the medicine, complained of a bad taste in her mouth and refused to take any more. Several weeks later she had a stroke. This had to be reported as an adverse event even though it was almost certain that it had nothing to do with the one pill she took. If there were more cases of strokes in the study group than in the control group, strokes would be classified as a side effect. This kind of process does not occur with herbal medicines or, I feel sure, we would be seeing a long list of side effects as well with herbal medicines.

> Coffee can give you insomnia, spicy foods can give you heartburn, beets can give your urine a red tint, and licorice can have a diuretic effect. I do not understand how some people can claim that natural products are completely free of side-effects.

Myth #5. Herbal medicine is more trustworthy than traditional medicine

Herbal remedies really increased in popularity in the 1980's and 1990's as a sort of backlash to conventional medicine. Conventional medicine was felt to be too expensive, too academic and arrogant, too dogmatic and controlled by Big Business with too much emphasis put on profits and the almighty buck. Herbal remedies became much more "politically correct". Being driven by money, conventional medicine was not to be trusted. The powerful pharmaceutical companies also had too much clout and influence in Washington with their powerful Lobbies.

This was also a time when technology itself was being questioned. We had just discovered a hole in the ozone layer that we had caused with our aerosols and CFC's. We had just become aware of global warming caused by our insatiable greed for energy and fossil fuels. We were wiping out ancient primordial rainforests with its multitude of bio-diversity all for the sake of "progress". We

SIMON FENG, M.D.

were getting too arrogant with our technology and destroying our whole planet in the process. How romantic the thought that herbal remedies could be earth-friendly, not motivated by greed and would be more affordable as well. The thought that maybe the ancients of China, Tibet or India knew things the arrogant medical societies didn't, was poetic justice. After all, when Nixon came back from China, there were all those images of surgeries performed completely under acupuncture anesthesia. Clearly, conventional western medicine did not know everything. If we were to live closer to the land with the innocence of the Native Americans, without the sins of the West, surely all would be well again. That was also the age of natural childbirth, the return of breast-feeding and the turn away from routine circumcision for boys.

I actually feel quite a bit of sympathy and agreement toward this philosophy and find the concept of returning to Nature just as appealing and idealistic. I agree that conventional medicine was guilty of many of the crimes it was accused of, such as arrogance and being profit-oriented. Very unfortunately however, herbal remedy companies have turned against this original philosophy. Again, I would like to state clearly that *I am not trying to attack herbal or alternative therapies, just the unethical practices of many of the companies that market these products*. These companies have now committed all the crimes that conventional medicine was ever guilty of. They are no longer earth-friendly because of all the farming land cleared for its cultivation as well as because of all the pesticide and herbicide use. Herbal medicines are now no longer cheap. The dietary supplement and herbal medicine industry has now become "Big Business" with a capital "B". As of 2003, it has been estimated to be a $17 billion a year industry. It has a very strong lobby in Washington. At least two times the FDA had tried to ban ephedra after athletes died from its use but was unsuccessful because of the strong influence of the lobby.

In my opinion, the herbal remedy market today is guilty of all the crimes that traditional medicine ever was before the days of FDA regulations. It is driven by greed for a fast profit. There is almost no accountability whatsoever. I believe that herbal remedies have betrayed the trust of its patients. Unscrupulous behavior is rampant. I had a colleague, a pediatrician, treating a child who was taking an "herbal" powder from China for asthma. The powder turned out to be prednisone powder, which had made the child suffer from steroid toxicity (known as Cushing's syndrome). This product was not labeled or tested properly and was not even really an herbal product.

> In my opinion, the herbal remedy market today is guilty of all the crimes that traditional medicine ever was before the days of FDA regulations.

In June 2003 FDA investigators found that two "nutritional supplements", *Vinarol* and *Viga*, marketed for "increasing desire, confidence and sexual performance" which were sold over the counter and through the internet contained the drug, Viagra (sildenafil)! This was not a contaminant but deliberately added to make the product work. It was not listed in the ingredients. To understand how horrible this is, many patients who were told by their physician they could not use Viagra because of a possible <u>fatal</u> interaction with their other medicines might resort to these herbal remedies as an alternative. Is this not unscrupulous? Yet, herbal medicines are becoming more and more mainstream and accepted. You can buy them at any drug store or supermarket. They are advertised on TV and giant billboards.

Many herbal preparations routinely contain five to ten different herbs in a concoction. Why? You would never accept a prescription from your MD for a pill containing that number of different drugs. Herbal preparations do not even have to list all their ingredients. They can classify them as "proprietary" which allows them to keep their ingredients secret, just as Kentucky Fried Chicken can keep its eleven spices and herbs "secret".

Myth #6. Herbal medications are backed up by research

It seems that whenever I hear an advertisement for herbal medications on radio or TV now, there is usually something to the effect that "studies show that…" or "clinically proven to…" I find this to be a very interesting phenomenon. Even though herbal remedies started out as a backlash to conventional medicine, they are trying more and more to sound like conventional medicines. If they say that "studies show" some effect or other, you need to find out who did these "studies". If they were done at a reputable University such as Harvard Medical School or at some well known clinic or hospital such as the Mayo Clinic, you can feel reasonably sure it was a legitimate study. If the study was done at "The Laboratory for the Advancement of Nutrition Therapy" (a fictitious name for a fictitious institute), you should be very skeptical. Where the study was published also makes a huge difference. If it were published in the Journal of the American Medical Association I would be far more ready to accept the results than if it were published in a newsletter printed by the herbal medicine company.

Conventional medicines that are controlled by the FDA are studied in research involving typically thousands, and sometimes tens of thousands, of patients in placebo-controlled double blind studies. (Double blind means that neither the doctor nor the patient knows if the patient is getting the real medicine or the placebo.) The studies quoted by herbal companies typically involve less than 50 or 100 patients, may not involve placebos and may not be double-blind. Results from this kind of research are not very reliable at all. If they quote a study, ask them how many patients were involved in this study.

Nutritional Supplements / Herbal Medications and the FDA

In order for a medication to be approved for sale in the United States, pharmaceutical companies must go through many steps to prove that the drug truly does what it says and that it is safe. This process often costs in the hundreds of millions of dollars to bring just one new drug to market. However, when it comes to nutritional supplements and herbal medications, **no proof is required** either that the product works or that it is safe, before it can be sold. If the FDA suspects the nutritional supplement to be unsafe, the FDA must prove it to be *harmful* in order to pull it from the market.

How did this state of affairs come into being? In 1958 the FDA was given the authority to regulate nutritional supplements just as it does with food or medications. It was only in 1994 that the FDA's authority over supplements was revoked when the Dietary Supplement Health and Education Act was passed with the support of lobbyists.

By calling them nutritional supplements, many chemical compounds can bypass the FDA's jurisdiction. Why is it that hormones such as growth hormone, melatonin or DHEA can be classified as nutritional supplements while other hormones such as insulin, thyroid hormone, estrogens and testosterones are regulated? Why are iron pills (prescribed for the treatment of anemia) such as ferrous sulfate regulated by the FDA but chromium picolinate is not? (Chromium picolinate is touted to treat a variety of problems from diabetes and high cholesterol to depression.)

Because herbal medicines are not answerable to the FDA or any other governmental agency, all kinds of claims of effectiveness can be made with little or no legitimate evidence. Products such as Human Growth Hormone claim to reverse aging, but there is little clinical evidence that it does so. Similarly, many herbal medicines that claim to grow hair probably do not do anything other than have a placebo effect. Many of the companies that produce these medications and make these claims are not afraid of being sued for false advertising or for health damages because most of the time they are limited liability companies. If they are ever sued successfully, they can close down and re-open next week as a different company. The big pharmaceutical companies cannot do this.

Herbal Remedies in General

While I believe that herbal remedies can make positive contributions in many areas other than weight loss, the present day herbal and nutritional supplement market needs to be approached with great caution. I would also like to say that conventional medicine has changed considerably in the intervening years. The medical profession is now far less arrogant, mostly because we have found too many times that we were wrong when we were sure that we were right. For decades we were sure that putting post-menopausal women on hormones was the right thing to do, but we now realize that we were wrong. We thought that the lower number of the blood pressure reading, the diastolic pressure, was the only important number, but we were wrong about that too. It was accepted dogma for a very long time that you do not put patients with heart failure on a class of medications called beta-blockers and that

SIMON FENG, M.D.

to do so was absolutely malpractice, but now we know we were sadly mistaken. There has been a real push in the past ten or fifteen years to practice evidence-based medicine. We are not perfect but we are improving.

It is my sincere wish that the nutritional supplement/herbal remedy industry can start becoming more accountable, more regulated and police-able. It needs an accrediting body that can monitor its practices, make sure claims are supportable and do proper, quality research. That way it can eventually become a full partner with conventional medicine. If my ranting here helps to push this along, I will be gratified. I believe that there is room for an ethical organization to rise to this challenge.

Am I suggesting that only fools would ever take an herbal medication? Not at all. All I ever ask of any medication is that it does what I want it to do without doing anything that I do not want it to do. If you take a blood pressure medication and it doesn't bring your blood pressure down, why are you taking it? If it brings your blood pressure down but it kills your sex life, it is still probably not the right medication for you.

You can apply the same criteria to herbal remedies. If you are currently taking something for your arthritis or your prostate, and the herbal medication is doing everything that you want without causing any problems, you do not have to change anything – but keep in mind the problems discussed above. If you have a medical problem and you are just not getting any satisfaction from conventional medicine, you can consider consulting an herbalist. Just as I would not advocate anyone take their friend's blood pressure medicine because it seemed to work for the friend, I would not advocate taking an herbal substance you know nothing about just because it seemed to work for your friend. If you do not have access to an herbalist, do some research on the internet, or better still, discuss it with your doctor or health care provider. Most of us today have access to reference material that at least have some information on potential side effects and precautions or contra-indications with the herbal medication, as well as possible interactions with other medications. Just do not assume herbs to be safe!

> All I ever ask of any medication, herbal or otherwise, is that it does what I want it to do, without doing anything that I do not want it to do.

As I am writing this book, I have a very dear friend who is fighting metastatic lung cancer. She has been through everything that Western Medicine has to offer. She has gone through surgery, chemotherapy and radiation therapy. She is currently in China, getting herbal medications at a facility that uses a combined approach using both western medicine and traditional Chinese medicine. This approach is helping her immensely. While it is not likely to cure her, it has helped her more than anything else. I was quite surprised to learn that she was getting herbal medicine extracts intravenously, but this is apparently not uncommon these days in China. (I must emphasize that these intravenous preparations were specifically formulated and sterilized for intravenous administration. Do not try other herbal medications intravenously!) She has my full blessing in using herbal medication, especially as her oncologist has told her there is not much left to offer her.

Herbal Weight Loss

While my comments on herbal remedies in general are true, I have seen no evidence for any safe and effective herbal weight loss. Most of the weight loss products available on the nutritional supplement/herbal market either contain amphetamine-like compounds, diuretics (they make you lose weight by losing fluid instead of fat), or laxatives. Many contain caffeine or caffeine-like substances that "stimulate" your metabolism. There is no miracle herb. Remember the adage, "If it sounds too good to be true, it probably is."

Metabolism Boosters

Another strategy that the herbal/nutritional supplement industry has adopted recently is the concept of metabolism boosters or "thermogenic agents". The idea is that these agents make your body burn up calories faster than normal and therefore "burn up fat". This concerns me very much. It is trying to make your body function in an

SIMON FENG, M.D.

abnormal way. It is like taking a car engine that should be idling at about 1000 rpm and making it idle at 2000 or 3000 rpm and driving it at two or three times the rate that it was designed to do. You can probably get away with it for a short period of time but it cannot be good for your car. Would you get into an elevator designed to hold eight people when it is crammed with 12 people? Would you get on board a plane that you knew was overloaded? When you force any machine (or your body) to run beyond what it was designed to do, there is a risk that things can go horribly wrong.

If you think that I am over-reacting, consider this: When athletes died from using ephedra, it was not the appetite suppressant effect that killed them but the metabolism-boosting action that made the heart race and put pressures on the heart past its tolerance. You need to exercise extreme caution with this strategy.

> When athletes died from using ephedra, it was not the appetite suppressant effect that killed them but the metabolism-boosting action that made the heart race and put pressures on the heart past its tolerance.

Chapter Four: The Medical Model of Obesity

"The aim of science is not to open the door to infinite wisdom,
But to set a limit to infinite error." – Bertolt Brecht (1898-1956)

Obesity as a Disease

There is a growing tendency to push obesity into a medical model, to be treated like an imbalance or a disease. There is no question that obesity is of extreme importance in medicine. It plays such a huge role in our physical and mental health. It becomes very easy to consider it as a disease. Obesity is an important factor in heart disease, the number one killer in America. It is a huge factor in a person developing diabetes. It has secondary effects on our health as well, by limiting our mobility and promoting a very sedentary lifestyle with all the negative impacts of poor cardiac conditioning. It also plays a very large role in wear-and-tear arthritis, further limiting our mobility.

Arguably more important than the effects on our physical health and life expectancy is the impact on our mental health and the quality of our life. Patients who are obese often suffer from poor self-esteem, feelings of worthlessness and depression. They often feel trapped. Even worse is the fact that these problems are all inter-related and tend to run in vicious cycles. When you have arthritis you aren't as active and gain weight easier, which makes the arthritis worse. If a patient is obese and suffers a heart attack, he or she is far more likely to feel that it was their fault, which can also leads to feelings of helplessness and hopelessness. This of course may lead to depression. Depression in turn can make many people eat and gain more weight, which further makes everything worse. So many of my obese patients feel hopeless, trapped and doomed. They resign themselves to poor health and give up. They no longer even try to take proper care of their diabetes, don't try to quit smoking and often do not take their medications the way they know they should. They feel that further health problems are unavoidable and resign themselves to whatever happens.

SIMON FENG, M.D.

Medical Treatment of Obesity

With all the impact that obesity has on health, it is understandable that we try to treat it as a disease. We all want to be able to measure it, define when it is abnormal, throw medications at it, and do surgery on it. We want to be able to blame it on our genes or on our environment. Concepts such as *Body Mass Index* and *Ideal Body Weight* are invented. We blame overweight problems on a slow metabolism, hypothyroidism, Cushing's syndrome, side effects of medicines, or other medical causes. There is a lot of money being spent on trying to find a "fat-gene" that explains why some people are overweight. There is a great deal of research going on to try to understand the biochemistry of satiety, involving hormones such as leptins and ghrelins and tumor necrosis factor-α. We are trying to understand what makes us feel full and what makes us hungry. We try to tweak the genes of laboratory mice to make them fat, and then try to give them medicines to make them thin again. Remind you of "Alice in Wonderland"?

The Holy Grail for researchers is to find the "magic bullet" pill that is going to control our appetites without any deleterious effects. Of course if this "magic bullet" is ever discovered, we will be able to treat obesity the same way that we treat high blood pressure or diabetes. It means that we can put patients on lifelong medications. Remember that in Chapter One I stated that permanent weight loss required a permanent change? Well, if we discovered such a medication, it would have to be a medication you take for the rest of your life and therefore would be a permanent change. There is obviously a very large incentive for pharmaceutical companies to find this "magic bullet", as the patient target base is the largest of any disease. If you figure in the long-term nature of the treatment, it would be easily the most successful drug of all time. When you consider the prevalence of depression and the amazing success of medications such as Prozac® and compare that with the prevalence of obesity you will stagger at how much money there is to be made.

Full-Service and Self-Service Medical Care

This is an explanation that I use to try to explain to patients about how they need to think about the treatment of their disease. I try to tell my patients that there are two kinds of medical treatments, Full-Service and Self-Service. If you have appendicitis, it is full-service. All you have to do is to lie there and let the doctors do everything. Similarly, if you need chemotherapy for cancer, it is all full-service.

On the other hand, if you are a diabetic, it really is self-service. You can't be taking a pill because I want you to, because your spouse wants you to, or because your mother wants you to. It only works well if you understand why you need to and you want to. When I leave the office at the end of the day, I leave behind all the diabetes, all the high blood pressures and all the high cholesterols. On the other hand, you own the disease and you get to carry it with you 24 hours a day, seven days a week, 52 weeks a year. I had a friend who was diabetic who would always tell me to turn my head when he wanted to eat something he shouldn't when I was present!

I tell my diabetics that it is their disease; the best I can possibly do is to be like a coach in the NBA. I am part of your team. I can set up plays and I can plan our strategy to take advantage of our strengths and their weaknesses, but guess what? I can't score a single point. I tell my diabetics that they are going to be living with their disease "…'til death do them part" so they might as well get to know their disease as well as they can.

The different types of treatment for obesity can also be separated into self-service and full-service. This is really important to understand because nothing happens if you are in the self-service line at the gas station expecting full-service. The only full-service treatment for obesity is bariatric surgery, which will be described later in this chapter.

Currently Available Pharmaceutical Treatments

Medications used to treat the overweight condition can be separated into several different categories:

1. Appetite suppressants
We have known since the 1960's that medications in the amphetamines class can all cause a reduction in appetite. There is no question that these medications can help the patient lose weight in the short term while the patient is taking the drugs.

SIMON FENG, M.D.

Unfortunately, all the weight comes back when the patient goes off the appetite suppressants. There was a school of thought in the medical field that patients should be treated with appetite suppressants on a long-term basis. The thought was that we treated high blood pressure like a chronic disease and did not just put them on blood pressure medicines for only three months. Similarly, obesity was a chronic disease and patients should also be put on appetite suppressants long-term.

There were two problems with this approach. First, studies show that after about six months, weight loss does not tend to continue but plateaus off. Often the weight started to climb again, even though the patient stayed on the appetite suppressants. This is unlike the case with blood pressure medications which still keep the blood pressure under control after many years. Second, long-term use of appetite suppressants may not be safe. The most infamous case was with Fen-Phen, the combination of two drugs, fenfluramine and phenteramine, which was found to be the most effective medication regimen for helping people lose weight but caused an unusual form of valvular heart disease. This was found to be due to the fenfluramine component and resulted in the withdrawal of fenfluramine and its cousin, dexfenfluramine, from the market.

Another drug used to suppress appetite is sibutramine, which has been shown to help in weight loss but the amount of weight lost was modest, usually in the neighborhood of ten pounds or so. It also can cause some blood pressure elevation.

2. Medical Mal-absorption

There is a drug known as orlistat that blocks the digestive enzymes from the stomach and pancreas that are responsible for the digestion of fats. These enzymes are lipases and the drug is known as a lipase-inhibitor. In theory, they prevent fat from being properly digested and absorbed. Sounds like you should be able to take one of these drugs then eat all the fatty foods that you love so much and never gain weight, right? Well, if you think that sounds too good to be true, you're right; it doesn't work like that. How it really works is that it blocks the absorption of only 15 % or so of the fats you eat, and the unabsorbed fats cause terrible side effects if you eat too much fat. The medication doesn't block enough fat absorption to make you lose weight but it does punish you for eating too much fatty food. If your diet contains more than 30% fat, you are going to get bad diarrhea and cramps. It really acts more like Antabuse®, which alcoholics take. Antabuse® makes you very nauseated if you drink alcohol after taking it, making it an effective deterrent. Orlistat can be useful to teach patients to eat the right kind of food. It punishes you for eating the wrong kinds of food. However, it is not the magic bullet. In my way of thinking, this drug can be very useful as a self-service tool, but is not effective as a full-service approach. If you think that all you need to do is to take this drug and you will lose weight, it won't work. Orlistat also does not help you to reduce the consumption or absorption of sugars and carbohydrates.

Ultimately, pharmaceutical methods of treating obesity are just not that effective at the present time. If there were a secret drug out there that really could make people lose weight safely and effectively, it would already have been used by all physicians everywhere, and obesity would not be the epidemic it is today.

Metabolic and Genetic Components of Obesity

There are definitely some patients who gain excess weight due to an abnormal metabolism or due to a genetic problem. Basically, people who have a genetic cause for their obesity are born with an inherited abnormal metabolism, whereas other people who are obese due to hypothyroidism or Cushing's syndrome developed an abnormal metabolism later in life. The genetic forms can be passed down to the next generation, but the acquired metabolic problems may not be. The question is really how much of a role these genetic/metabolic abnormalities have played in the obesity epidemic.

We often see obese parents with obese children, making it easy to assume that it is genetic. It may even be more polite and politically correct to think that. However, as we know, parents pass a whole lot more down to their offspring than just genetic material. We also give them coping mechanisms, prejudices, mannerisms and, oh yes, attitudes. We know that children growing up in a home where there is domestic violence are far more likely to engage in domestic violence. If you have a parent in professional sports, it is more likely

SIMON FENG, M.D.

that you will take up the same sport. Think also about the Kennedy clan and politics. Another example would be religion: if your parents were Catholics, it is much more likely that you would be Catholic as well. Similarly, if your parents were Buddhists or Muslims, your chances of being one as well are much higher.

I think that people with weight problems would like to believe they have an inherited genetic cause for their obesity. That means that it is really not their fault. You have no control over the eye color you were born with, and it is a lot healthier for your self-esteem to believe that you also cannot help being overweight.

Well, if you had no choice of the genes you got from your parents, you also had no choice in the habits, lifestyles or attitudes you got from your parents. However, while you cannot change your genes, there is at least a possibility that you can change your bad habits, lifestyles and unhealthy attitudes!

> If you had no choice of the genes you got from your parents, you also had no choice in the habits, lifestyles or attitudes you got from your parents.

How much of a role does genetics play in obesity? I believe the role is a very minor one. Scientists and pharmaceutical companies would like to believe that genes play a huge role because that would mean there was potential to invent a drug to treat this genetic or metabolic flaw (and make lots of money). It is this mind-set that has largely determined the direction of research into obesity. When scientists discover that obese people have different levels of hormones such as leptins, that they have different degrees of insulin sensitivity, does it mean that these change are responsible for the weight gain? Could it mean instead that obesity caused the differences?

I believe that there are rare cases of obesity due to genetic factors, but the "Rank and File" overweight person does not have any genetic or metabolic disorder. In support of this viewpoint, I would like to point out that obesity is on the rise all over America (see Chapter Two). Genetic diseases tend to remain fairly constant in the population. The prevalence of cystic fibrosis or sickle cell disease does not change much unless the racial mix of the population changes. Also, obesity rates among Asians in America are much higher than the rates in Asia, even though the genes are the same. Germans in Germany are not as fat as Germans living in America. I believe the situation is the same for Africans in Africa versus African Americans. Genetics? I don't see it. Genetics determines fat distribution patterns so that some people deposit more fat on their necks while others deposit more fat on their hips. Some people may even have a genetic predisposition to gain weight more easily, but genetics alone cannot explain the epidemic of obesity.

There was a very interesting study done in Denmark in the late-1980's that looked at how obesity was related to genetics. The study looked at people adopted in childhood and compared their adult weights with those of their adoptive parents and their biological parents. The results showed that being thin had a genetic component but obese biological parents did not correlate to obese children.

The other area of research that shows the limited role genetics plays in obesity involves the Pima Indians in Arizona, who have the highest rates of obesity and diabetes of any racial group in the world. If any group has a genetic cause for their obesity it would be this group. Yet, if you compare the Pima Indians of Arizona with the Pima Indians of Mexico, you'll find that the Mexican Pima Indians are not obese and do not have the prevalence of diabetes of their American counterparts. Furthermore, if you compare Pima Indians in Arizona before and after World War II, you will find similarly that the obesity and diabetes rates only went up after World War II. While it remains possible that Pima Indians have a genetic weakness to weight gain, the prevalence of obesity among the Pima Indians of Arizona is much more due to sociological and cultural factors than genetic factors.

Even if you have a genetic predisposition to weight gain, it doesn't doom you to that fate. There have been very good studies done involving identical twins separated at birth. These twins share exactly the same genetic material but grew up in different environments. These types of studies have been instrumental in understanding the roles that genetics and environment play in many disorders. We know that if one twin was an alcoholic, there was a 50% chance that the other twin will also be an alcoholic. This tells us that alcoholism can have a genetic component but it also tells us that we are not doomed by our genes. This should also have been evident in that alcoholics can recover from their addiction. Similarly, even if you have a genetic component to your obesity, you are not doomed to it.

> Even if you have a genetic component to your obesity, you are not doomed to it.

Short Comings of the Medical Model

I actually think that the medical model (treating obesity as a disease) is quite an improvement and advance from the old model, where obesity was viewed as a weakness and/or laziness. It was viewed as the sentence for the crime of greed, the punishment for the sin of gluttony. It was the consequence of the weakness of poor self-discipline and the result of laziness. Another very good effect of the medical model of obesity is that it is becoming much more acceptable for patients to come in seeking help for their weight problems. It is still more embarrassing to come in to see the doctor for weight problems than for hypertension but it is probably less embarrassing than asking for Viagra®.

The main problem that I see with the present medical model is that it assumes that the root cause (or etiology) of obesity is caloric imbalance. Hence, all the treatment has been directed either at trying to reduce the caloric intake or trying to increase the caloric expenditure through exercise. Even where the medical model looks for an underlying cause for the caloric imbalance, it only looks into the biological basis with fat genes and hormones. My main thesis is that the over-consumption of calories is itself only a symptom of underlying sociological and cultural attitudes toward food that must be addressed for successful long-term weight loss. Treating the symptom only is not very successful. If you treat a patient with pneumonia with cough-suppressants and acetaminophen for the fever, it is not enough. Similarly, we must look at how and why we became overweight.

> The over-consumption of calories is in itself only a symptom of deeper underlying unhealthy attitudes toward food that must be addressed for successful long-term weight loss.

Bariatric Surgery

The term bariatric comes from the Greek word, "*baros*" for heavy, and bariatric surgery is surgery to treat obesity. This is the short cut. This is the solution that bypasses all the socio-cultural causes of obesity and it needs to be mentioned here. It is the ultimate last resort. It is definitely not for everyone, but it can also do the job when nothing else can.

Over the past 30 odd years different surgical strategies have been tried to induce weight loss. Some of these surgical strategies included gastric stapling, putting constricting rings around the stomach and various ways of re-arranging the anatomy of the digestive tract. These surgeries either limit the amount of food you can eat or greatly reduce the ability of the body to absorb nutrients (calories) from the food in the digestive tract. Many of these have been unsuccessful at best and disastrous at worst. Many of the gastric rings eroded into the stomach, caused perforations, or slipped further down toward the small intestine and became ineffective. Some of the surgical rearrangements led to what are known as blind-loops, which got into trouble with infections and bacterial overgrowth. There were complications such as "dumping syndromes" when the body would react to a larger meal or to too much sugar with abdominal cramps, diarrhea and sometimes hot flushes. There were also problems with mal-absorption. Many of these procedures eventually had to be reversed.

The procedure that proved to be the most successful long term, with manageable complications, was gastric by-pass. In this procedure, which is the most popular today, most of the stomach is separated and usually cut off. The functioning part of the stomach that is left is only about the size of a golf ball and it is hooked up directly to the small bowel further downstream. How the surgery works is that in the first place you can't eat very much at all, maybe three or four ounces. It is still possible to gain weight by eating or drinking small amounts of food or drink all day long. The surgery also works by limiting the amount of sugar you can take in, as too much sugar causes a dumping syndrome. Malnutrition needs to be addressed with long-term vitamins.

SIMON FENG, M.D.

There is no question that this kind of bariatric surgery can be very successful. For many people it is the only therapy that seems to work. The biggest reason for the appeal and success of bariatric surgery, in my opinion, is that it is the only full-service approach to obesity. Everything else requires some degree of work and commitment on the part of the patient. The problems with this surgery include all the risks of surgery and anesthesia. There is a definite mortality rate from the surgery. The larger the patient, the higher the risks of complications. For the really large patient over 500 pounds, the risks of dying from the surgery or from post-surgical complications may outweigh the benefits of the surgery.

> The biggest reason for the appeal and success of bariatric surgery, in my opinion, is that it is the only full-service approach to obesity.

There is also the problem of getting insurance to pay for the surgery, although it seems to be approved as often as it is disallowed. Clearly, this approach can be successful but is not for everyone. It is also not universally available.

Bariatric surgery is clearly not for the merely overweight or even the mildly obese. While obesity is defined as a BMI of over 30, obesity is also categorized into Class 1 (BMI of 30-35), Class 2 (BMI of 35-40) and Class 3 (BMI of greater than 40). Class 3 obesity is also known as *morbid obesity*. In general, bariatric surgery may be justified for those with Class 3 obesity, but this is only a guideline. Many surgeons will consider someone in Class 2 or possibly even Class 1 obesity for surgery if they have other life-threatening health problems, such as diabetes, that are made worse by the obesity. Age is also a factor, as few surgeons would responsibly perform surgery on someone over the age of 70 or on a teenager of 15.

One other word of caution: With the recent increase in the popularity of bariatric surgery, there have been reports of some surgeons performing these surgeries now who were not properly trained in bariatric medicine. Due to the fact that these surgeries rearrange the anatomy, the body functions in an abnormal manner after surgery. Complications such as mal-absorption, malnutrition, liver problems and dumping syndromes all need to be managed. The dosages of many medicines such as blood pressure medications or diabetic medications may need to be changed drastically immediately after surgery. Patients need to be followed up for years after the surgery. They can run into problems with iron-deficiency, vitamin deficiencies and osteoporosis.

Bariatric surgery is best performed as part of a multi-disciplinary approach involving surgeons, dietitians and psychologists. Make sure that the surgeon has a special interest in the treatment of obesity and has been properly trained. There is much more to the properly-trained bariatric surgeon than merely the technical ability to do the surgery.

> There is much more to the properly-trained bariatric surgeon than merely the technical ability to do the surgery.

Chapter Five: Medical Reasons for Weight Gain

« Felix qui potuit rerum cognoscere causas » "Lucky is he who has been able to understand the causes of things." – Virgil 70-19 BC

There are quite a few conditions that not infrequently cause varying degrees of weight gain. Sometimes these are the primary reason why someone became overweight in the first place; however, sometimes they are merely factors that complicate any attempts at weight loss. Any wish for successful weight loss needs to take these conditions into consideration.

Hypothyroidism

In my experience, hypothyroidism can be an important factor in weight loss but is not usually responsible for gross obesity. If you have experienced significant unexplained weight gain over the past year or so, it is imperative that you get your thyroid status checked. If on the other hand you have been overweight for the last 20 years, it is quite unlikely that hypothyroidism is the culprit.

If depression or fatigue plays a big role in your weight gain you also need to get your thyroid checked. It is very important to realize that on occasion the main complaint for some people who have hypothyroidism is depression. Also, if you have trouble losing weight you should make sure that you are not deficient in thyroid hormone. However, in general, even though everyone blames a slow metabolism for their weight, an abnormal metabolism is probably not that big a factor in most cases.

Cushing's Syndrome

This is a condition that happens when the body has too much cortisone, either from overactive adrenal glands or from medications (steroids) taken long term for various medical reasons. It is not nearly as common as hypothyroidism but is always mentioned as a cause of obesity. It can present with a variety of different symptoms but the most common are central obesity (the arms and legs remain thin while the fat is distributed around the trunk, face and abdomen), high blood pressure and diabetes. If you have these symptoms, don't panic – it is still unlikely that you have Cushing's syndrome; however, it might be worthwhile to get it checked out.

Post-Partum Weight Gain

Many women have told me that they never had a weight problem until after childbirth. They believe that it is some sort of hormonal change that caused this weight gain. Instead, I believe that it is because their lifestyles changed drastically. It is of course true that we encourage a minimum weight gain of 25 pounds with a normal term pregnancy, which is not always easy to lose after childbirth. Nevertheless, it must not be forgotten how much your life changes after your first baby. First of all, if there is any degree of post-partum depression it makes weight loss much harder. Even in the absence of post-partum depression there are still profound changes. People without children of their own often think they understand what having children must be like. One of my favorite phrases that I say to them is, "Trying to explain children to people without children is harder than trying to explain sex to a virgin!" Parents all understand this. You don't sleep the same way again for a very long time, maybe forever. For the first several weeks after childbirth you are functioning in a completely different mode from how you have ever functioned before. For the first time in your life you have total and complete responsibility for another human being that is, unbelievably, your child. The whole experience of childbirth itself has been awe-inspiring and left you hurting and tired. You have been used to eating for two and you are in a mode of thought where your personal appearance is of necessity of lesser importance. Suffice it to say that the post-partum period has an abundance of reasons that account for the weight gain without invoking any mysterious hormonal change that forever altered the body. Motherhood also frequently involves the preparation of food and drink and snacks, all of which may be too accessible.

Once the weight gain has set in, it often triggers one of the unhealthy eating patterns we will discuss in Chapter Seven. Treatment will be directed at the unhealthy eating patterns rather than addressing some mysterious metabolic change that happened after childbirth many years ago.

Chronic Fatigue

Many chronic medical problems can manifest as chronic fatigue. These include different kinds of inflammatory arthritis, chronic low back pain or other chronic disabilities, fibromyalgia, and others. At any rate, chronic fatigue can predispose to weight gain by several mechanisms. There is reduced activity and with that comes reduced caloric requirement. There is also possibly some degree of comfort eating.

Treatments for these problems are sometimes quite difficult and not always satisfactory. I want to word this next part very carefully as what I want to say may be misunderstood very easily. If you find yourself getting upset, give me the benefit of the doubt and read on through.

There is considerable overlap between fibromyalgia, chronic fatigue, irritable bowel syndrome and some degree of depression. I am not trying to say they are all caused by depression. In the case of irritable bowel syndrome, this might be a little easier to understand because we know that many of the same neurotransmitters in the brain, such as serotonin, are also found in the gut. This is why so many of the anti-depressants that we use have some degree of gastrointestinal side effects. It is not too far of a mental leap to hypothesize that when a "chemical imbalance" occurs in the brain, it may also occur in the gut. I am not sure if some similar kind of chemical overlap is also involved in fibromyalgia or not. What I do know is that anti-depressants are often useful in the treatment of these disorders. In fact, I know of a physician who goes as far as to say, "I have never known a patient with fibromyalgia to do well in the absence of anti-depressants." Most patients with these problems will also tell you that their symptoms all seem to get worse when they are under stress.

What I am saying is not that these chronic diseases are synonymous with depression and "all in your head". Better perhaps to say that there is a link between mind and body, and people with

SIMON FENG, M.D.

these medical problems seem to have a closer link between mind and body.

The closest example that I can think of to illustrate the use of anti-depressants in these problems is the fact that we use blood pressure medications such as propranolol to treat migraine headaches. We can also use anti-epileptic medications to treat migraines. It is not because we think that their migraines are really seizures or caused by high blood pressure. However, the receptors that propranolol works on are on the blood vessels, and migraines are caused by blood vessels going into spasm in the brain.

Sleep Apnea

This is frequently undiagnosed and can be a very significant health problem. In brief, this is a condition where a person's breathing is compromised at nighttime during sleep. Usually this is the result of a relatively small airway. The tongue falls back during sleep and obstructs the breathing. The patient can go for as long as two minutes without breathing, and finally wakes up very lightly (not enough so that he or she can remember waking up) but can do so sometimes over 100 times in a night. This results in very fragmented sleep, never getting into proper deep sleep. The patient wakes up in the morning feeling tired, what we call non-restorative sleep. They complain of tiredness all day and fall asleep at the drop of a hat. In severe cases, they may fall asleep while driving or while waiting for traffic lights to change.

The relationship between sleep apnea and weight gain can be a little bit of the "chicken or egg" situation. There is no question that sleep apnea can cause fatigue, which can lead to significant weight gain. However, when a person is significantly overweight, the airway is almost always smaller and blocks off much more easily and can either cause obstructive sleep apnea or make it worse. If there is any degree of sleep apnea that warrants treatment, it needs to be addressed.

Effects of Medications

There are many different medications sometimes associated with weight gain. Most of the medications that cause weight gain only cause mild to modest weight gain, but there are a few that can cause marked weight gain. In order for the weight gain to be considered significant, patients need to gain 7% or more of their original weight. This does not mean that the patient won't be upset if he or she gains "only" 5% of body weight.

The more important consideration to me is whether or not the weight gain is likely to be limited. Most medications that cause weight gain, such as birth control pills, may result in something like a five-pound weight gain, which then usually levels off. If a patient gains 30 pounds on birth control pills, I would highly suspect some other cause. On the other hand, there are some medications that can on occasion cause marked weight gain of 30 pounds or more.

If you feel that some of your weight gain is secondary to medications, it is essential that you discuss this with your physician. Often there is an alternative medication that won't be as problematic. If there is absolutely no other choice and the condition must be treated, we can consider adding another medication which may help to counteract this weight gain. Do not stop your medications without discussing it with your doctor or health care provider.

Smoking Cessation

The other time when weight gain can become problematic is when people try to quit smoking. I strongly believe that this weight gain is secondary to one or more unhealthy eating patterns coming into play. Often the person trying to quit starts to snack or drink a lot of soft drinks to compensate for not smoking. Eating out of boredom may play a role, as the ex-smoker is constantly looking for something to do with his or her hands. Comfort eating can also be involved. These specific eating patterns are discussed further in Chapter Seven.

What can be done is to make sure you use some of the aids out there to help you quit, such as nicotine patches or inhalers, or

SIMON FENG, M.D.

perhaps Zyban®. It is really important to quit smoking. Luckily, most of the time weight gain with smoking cessation is limited to five or ten pounds before it stabilizes, and often with time this weight is lost again. If you are careful not to let one of the unhealthy eating patterns kick in, you should be able to avoid marked weight gain. A temporary weight gain of five to ten pounds is, I believe, a small price to pay to rid yourself of cigarettes. Just remember that it is not worthwhile to start smoking again after you have successfully quit and now gained your five or ten pounds needlessly.

Serious Illness

Oftentimes significant weight gain follows a serious bout of illness or injury. This may represent a bad motor vehicle accident, a work-related back injury or a severe bout of arthritis. There are several mechanisms by which the weight gain occurs.

Illness or injury causes very significant changes in the patient's lifestyle.
A serious knee injury that sidelines the athlete for a prolonged period of time is an example of this. Any serious illness that requires prolonged bed rest for recovery also can fall into this category.

Depression may set in
This is especially true when the injury or illness affects the ability to work and earn a living.
Injuries or illnesses that cause permanent disability are very prone to complications of depression. These include spinal cord injuries, injuries that cause the loss of a limb or the loss of sight, and medical diseases such as severe arthritis. Realizing that you are never going to get better is a hard pill to swallow and depression sets in easily.

Medications may cause weight gain as a side effect
This category has been discussed earlier in the chapter.

<u>Combination of the above</u>
Serious illnesses frequently cause weight gain in more than one way. Severe arthritis sometimes requires treatment with steroids, so the patient has all three mechanisms going on at the same time: steroids make them gain weight, their lifestyle is forever changed and depression is not uncommon.

Summary

There are also a host of very rare conditions such as hypothalamic syndromes where the part of the brain that controls appetite is selectively destroyed by injury or stroke. This chapter lists medical causes of obesity, but the point is that they account for only a small percentage of the overweight. I have found quite a few overweight people who were hypothyroid but their weight did not return to normal when we fixed their thyroid problem, unless they were only mildly overweight. Nevertheless, it is very important to diagnose their hypothyroidism as I believe they cannot lose weight successfully if we do not take care of their thyroid.

I believe the overwhelming amount of overweight is due to other factors discussed in the next section.

SECTION THREE

A New Viewpoint

Chapter Six: Unhealthy Attitudes

"I never feel lonely in the kitchen. Food is very friendly." – Julia Child

Section Two of this book (Chapters 3 to 5) dealt with the medical model and the current ways of thinking about and treating obesity. In this Section, I would like to put forth my thoughts on obesity. While these are original thoughts, I believe the truth of these viewpoints will prove to be self-evident.

I have stated in the previous chapters that we need to look past caloric imbalance to find the true cause(s) of obesity and the overweight condition. While there is no question that caloric imbalance is the mechanism by which people become overweight, I strongly believe that there are real reasons why one person develops this caloric imbalance when another does not. If we could discover why this is so, maybe we could reverse it. In the course of my 19 years of practice as a family physician, I have known a great number of people. I know that for any obese person, I can find you another who is the same age, same height, same race, same state of health, same educational achievement level, same background and under the same amount of stress, yet is not overweight. Some people blame their weight problems on the fact that they are unhappy or depressed, but similarly, I can find you someone else who is just as unhappy but is not overweight. What makes one person overweight but not the other? Why does one person develop a caloric imbalance that the other does not? While there certainly could be genetic or metabolic causes of obesity, I am of the very firm belief that they play a relatively minor role.

I have long observed sociological and cultural differences in the rates of obesity, and the research bears this out. Studies show that rates of obesity vary considerably depending on one's race, gender and, very interestingly, one's level of educational achievement and socioeconomic status. It was thoughts like these that lead to my theories about the role of sociology in the cause of obesity. My hope was that this line of inquiry would lead beyond the "How's" of obesity to the "Why's" of obesity. Once we knew why people become overweight, we might be able to formulate treatments that actually make sense.

SIMON FENG, M.D.

My explorations into the sociological causes of obesity led me to two different types of abnormalities that I now consider to be the main causes of the current obesity epidemic:

1. Unhealthy Attitudes toward Food
2. Unhealthy Eating Patterns.

In this chapter, I wish to explore in greater detail the relationship between culture, sociology and obesity, which I consider to have given rise to what I call "Unhealthy Attitudes toward Food". In the next chapter, I try to show how these unhealthy attitudes manifest themselves as "Unhealthy Eating Patterns" that lead to the caloric imbalance which result in abnormal weight gain.

The Sociological/Cultural Basis of Obesity

I do not believe it is a coincidence that the past decades which saw the biggest change in American society also saw the dramatic increase in obesity. Indeed, I believe that it is precisely the changes in society over the past 50 years or so that are largely responsible for the marked increase in obesity. I believe that the underlying causes of obesity are sociological or cultural, and this is where we ultimately need to intervene.

As a sign of how much society has changed in the past 100 years, it has been noted that 100 years ago, life expectancy in North America was only 40 years. The other factoid that really surprised me was that 100 years ago there were more people living in Alabama than there were in the entire state of California.

How has societal change affected our waistlines and how does it account for the epidemic of obesity? There are five main socio-cultural reasons that I have identified to explain the epidemic of obesity in America.

Changes in Social Structure

Society has changed markedly since the end of The Second World War. America has become more prosperous, and with prosperity have come higher expectations. People have become far more mobile because of better transportation, better vehicles and better highways. There have been marked changes in the structure of the family. Often child care has become a problem, with no grandparents or other family around. Frequently both parents have had to work, leaving very little time for the preparation of meals. The prevalence of divorce and family break-up in today's society is much higher, significantly changing family dynamics. Non-traditional families have become much more common.

Because most of these changes put more stresses on the family, time for the preparation of food became harder to set aside. With all of these changes, processed and pre-packaged foods have found amazing success. The impact of TV dinners on American society has been significant. Processed foods came to be viewed as progress, even glamorous. Tang®, a crystallized instant orange drink powder, was all the rage in the 1960's because that was what the astronauts drank. It was felt to be better than orange juice. Baby food had to come in a little glass jar with the picture of a cute baby on it. New parents were intimidated by the thought of preparing baby foods themselves that may not be sterile enough, undercooked, overcooked or had too much salt.

Into this atmosphere, fast food just came naturally. When the first fast food restaurants opened for business, it was certainly quite exciting and felt like real progress. With the popularity of pre-packaged foods, sodas soon came in single serving bottles, candy bars and potato chips joined in and a good profit was enjoyed by all. All this introduced sugar into the American diet to an extent never seen before. There is far more sugar in the average American diet today with doughnuts, candy, desserts and sodas.

Changes in the Content of the Modern Diet

The North American diet has been changing drastically over the past half century, and I don't think that too many people would contest that this plays a large part in the epidemic of obesity that we have seen. A much higher percentage of our food intake now comprises processed foods instead of home-cooked. All this processed food has a lot more sugar, salt and fat than in days past.

SIMON FENG, M.D.

Obviously, these changes need to be addressed if we wish to avoid weight problems.

The answer may be for fast food outlets to start offering more healthy alternatives. To a large extent I find that this is already starting to be seen, with McDonald's now offering salads and Arby's offering Market Fresh Sandwiches, as well as newer regional fast food restaurants that offer healthier alternatives. However, I would like to point out that people without weight problems also eat at fast food restaurants without any major problems with their weights.

I think people without weight problems tend to eat far less doughnuts, candy, cookies, potato chips and chocolates than overweight people. There is no question in my mind that these items need to be permanently limited if any permanent weight loss is desired. It does not mean that you can't ever have another cookie or potato chip. What it does mean is that you can't be eating any of these sweet treats on a daily or regular basis. If you really enjoy cookies, as I do, you just need to make sure you only eat them once in a while and not more than one, perhaps two, at a time. You simply can't sit down and eat a whole box of them at one sitting. This is not an issue for people without weight problems. If you can't just eat one cookie and stop, you may have an unhealthy attitude toward food and/or unhealthy eating pattern that we need to address, which is the subject of these next two chapters.

> If you can't just eat one cookie and stop, you may have an unhealthy attitude toward food and/or unhealthy eating pattern that we need to address

More Sedentary Lifestyle

There is no disagreement that both children and adults are much more sedentary today than in the past. This started with the popularity of movies and television, and continued with computer games. I must point out that sedentary activity has always existed in the way of board games, chess and reading. The big difference is that in the past, few kids would be reading at the expense of playing in the playground or swimming. Now, kids are content to play video games for hours or watch TV *all day*. For the adults, TV and the internet are big causes of a sedentary lifestyle. One difference between these two activities that should be mentioned is that working on the computer requires the use of one or both hands, and so people are less likely to eat while doing this activity as opposed to watching TV.

The other big difference in our level of activity has been the introduction of labor-saving devices and power tools as well as convenient services. Motor vehicles mean that we do not expend the calories walking as we did in the past. Washing machines, power saws, self-propelled lawn-mowers and automated car washes all save us a lot of energy (also known as calories). Not only are we saving calorie expenditure at home but also at work in factories, mines and farms, where there are power tools to save us labor. The only way a lot of us break a sweat nowadays is when we go to the gym.

Changes in Ideal Body Image

With the advent of the movie industry and the changing of role models into glamorous stereotypical sex symbols/celebrities, such as movie stars, music stars, athletes and models, the standard of beauty has changed dramatically. Never has sex-appeal been so important, and sex-appeal today is not about being overweight. Our ideal image of what constitutes a sexy body has changed gradually. When you look at nude paintings by the great artists of the Renaissance era, you will notice that they were usually plump, as that was the standard of beauty at that time. Not any more. I have seen statistics that show that winners of the Miss America pageant have been getting leaner and leaner as the years go by. Even Marilyn Monroe would be considered plump by today's standards. Perceptions of being overweight often lead to feelings of shame and inadequacy, as well as to lower self-esteem. Instead of motivating the person to lose weight, more often than not it leads instead to a host of compensatory behaviors that contribute to and exacerbate the problem. I believe that these compensatory behaviors often lead to many unhealthy eating patterns, which will be discussed in the next chapter.

SIMON FENG, M.D.

Unhealthy Attitudes

I believe that one of the biggest reasons that people gain weight is not what they eat but rather why and how they eat, and that the main reason for obesity may be an unhealthy attitude toward food. We no longer eat for sustenance. Food is Recreation; it is fun to eat everything from candy to pizza. Food is Reward; we are rewarded by food for our hard work and for our good behavior. We treat our kids to ice cream when they have been good or bring home a good report card. Food is Love; if you love someone, you feed that person. We eat when we are lonely; we eat when we are with friends. We feast when we are happy and we binge when we feel bad. Our parents tell us that we must never waste food because there are starving kids in Somalia. We go to "All You Can Eat Buffets" and eat all we can to get "our money's worth". We do not eat until we are no longer hungry but instead we eat until we are uncomfortably full.

Aversion to Wasting Food

Let us deal with some of these issues starting with overeating. Why do we overeat? How do we decide on how much food we are going to be eating at the next meal? For many of us, how much we eat at a meal depends on how much food our mothers, spouses or waiters put on the plate in front of us. We always finish whatever food is in front of us. If we leave anything it is usually a few vegetables or a bit of potato - something that is not considered to be expensive or wasteful to throw away. The reason for this is that we are taught from a very young age not to waste food, that there are children starving in the world. Waste is a sin. I remember my own mother relating to me what her mother used to tell her, "If you throw away money, somebody will pick it up and find a use for it but if you throw away food, it will forever be wasted." I used to reply, "Either it's going to waste or it's going to waist!"

I never understood this. How does my finishing my plate after I am already full help a starving child in Ethiopia? Does that child feel less hungry if I overeat? If there is waste, it is not because I did not eat it but because it should never have been bought or prepared in the first place. If I throw away the food it will harm nobody, but if I eat it someone (me) will be harmed.

This aversion toward wasting food is universal in all cultures that I am aware of. This aversion is also logical because in most areas of the world there is true poverty and having enough money to buy food is a constant struggle. It is heartbreaking to realize that people are still dying of hunger in the world. This is simply not the case in North America. When was the last time you heard of somebody dying of hunger in America or Canada? If someone did die of hunger in America it would be shocking news in every newspaper. On the other hand, when somebody dies of hunger in Bangladesh or Somalia it may not even be reported in the local newspaper. Up to the very recent past, famines were frequent and recurrent. This is still the case in many parts of the world. But when was the last famine in America?

I guess that America is a victim of its own success in this regard. Nobody really remembers the last famine in America. It is probably not a coincidence that America is at the same time the most prosperous nation as well as the most obese. It is not necessarily the American culture that is causing the epidemic of obesity so much as the culture of prosperity. As other industrialized nations become more prosperous they may have their own problems with obesity. The very strong aversion to wasting food served us very well and had real survival value when we faced occasional food shortages and famines. In today's society, it now contributes in no small degree to our health problems and mortality.

Interestingly, as nations become more developed, industrialized and prosperous, their levels of obesity rise. Within developed countries however, obesity is a much greater problem among the lower socioeconomic strata and those with lower educational achievement. In other words, in Third World countries, it is the rich who are fat, but in America it is the poor who are at most risk of being obese. This may go against intuition, as our classic tales of "A Christmas Carol", "Oliver Twist" and others all equate poverty with hunger. Nevertheless, it is true that the poor in America are at greater risk of obesity.

Quantumization of Food

The other phenomenon that has contributed to the weight problem is what I call the "quantumization of food". What I mean by

SIMON FENG, M.D.

this is that foods now come in fixed "quanta" better known as the serving size. One big advantage that the traditional Chinese way of eating has is that there is no fixed amount of food that you are supposed to eat. All the dishes are put in the middle of the dining table while everyone has his or her own bowl of rice. Every person then picks whatever food he or she wants from the middle of the table. On the other hand, in America we are served a given portion that can't be refused. All kinds of food now come in specific serving sizes, such as one doughnut, one breakfast bar, one bag of chips. This quantumization of food is really for the benefit of the food industry as it is a lot easier to package and more profitable to sell. But think about this: two men go to a fast-food outlet and both order the same meal package even though one may weigh 190 pounds while the other weighs 160 pounds. Surely one is either getting too much or the other is not getting enough.

This would not be so bad except for the fact that we are conditioned against throwing away or wasting food. No restaurant would want to be known as one that has serving sizes that are too small. The portion sizes keep getting bigger until we could not possibly finish it all, but because of our aversion to throwing away food, we must necessarily overeat. This phenomenon has led to the culture of "super-sizing". You can get a better "deal" on the meal if you order the super-sized package. If you did not get the extra-large version and found that you were still hungry after eating the regular meal-deal, it would cost you a lot more to get more food. Better be safe and order the super-sized version, right? Of course once you have ordered the extra-large meal, you have to finish it to get your money's worth!

The other big problem with serving sizes is the fact that individual portion sizes are getting larger all the time. I remember a time when the regular drink serving was 8 oz. Now you can go to a gas station and find that the small size is 16 oz, the medium is 20 oz while the big daddy is 32 oz!

Unhealthy Attitudes are Learned in Childhood

Part of the problem is that this pattern of eating is deeply ingrained in us. We were told from the time we were very young that we were not allowed to leave the table until we had eaten all our greens or meat. We are taught to ignore our bodily signals that tell us that we are full. We are taught to keep eating even though our bodies tell us we shouldn't eat any more. If we are good and do that, by golly, we get rewarded with dessert! Then 20 or 30 years later, we wonder why we have a weight problem. We spend millions of dollars in research to find a chemical compound that will tell us that we are full while we have been spending all our lives teaching our children to ignore those same signals. Doesn't that strike you as just a little crazy? Observe how children without weight problems eat. As soon as they are full, they want to leave the table. If you take them to an "all-you-can-eat buffet", they don't really eat all that more than they normally do. If you give them a tubful of ice cream they don't just keep eating. However, if we keep teaching them to ignore their bodily signals they will soon learn to overeat. Even more than wanting to help people to lose weight, I want this society to learn how *not* to teach our children to have these wrong and unhealthy attitudes toward food, perpetuating the problem into the next generation. If you can't unlearn your behavior, at least let us not pass on the unhealthy attitudes to the children.

As I have previously mentioned, we pass more down to our children than just genetic material; we pass down many of our attitudes and viewpoints. We have no choice in the genes that we pass to our children, but we can control the unhealthy attitudes now that we are aware of them.

Food as Reward/Entitlement

Food is frequently used as a form of reward in childhood. We promise to take children for ice cream if they are good. When we take them to the doctor for immunizations, they get candy. Dessert is the reward for "eating properly" (or is it "eating improperly"?). Unfortunately, this attitude persists into adulthood and becomes perhaps one of the most important of the unhealthy attitudes. Whenever an overweight person has had a very tough day at work, he or she comes home and wants to reward himself or herself with something tasty. It is perhaps reward for putting up with a bad boss and not quitting. Food is often the reward for a hard day at work (except that every day at work may be considered a hard day). After spending all day doing what your boss wants, what your kids need and what you have to do, there is a sense of entitlement that now, "I deserve to do something for myself!" Food is too easy to use as entitlement.

One of the most powerful aspects of this feeling of entitlement is that it allows a person to rationalize behavior that he or she knows is wrong. This, I believe, is possibly the main cause of comfort eating. Comfort eaters know that they are doing something that they really should not be doing. They may even realize that they are going to regret it later, but they do it anyway. Why? Because in their minds, they deserve the reward of food.

> One of the most powerful aspects of this feeling of entitlement is that it allows a person to rationalize behavior that he or she knows is wrong.

If my understanding of Human Nature is not incorrect, I believe that this sense of entitlement plays a very big role in causing obesity in those who perceive themselves to be underprivileged. Many people who feel that they have not had a fair shake in life feel entitled to take some form of enjoyment in life. Food fits the bill easily for many. Food is cheap entertainment that is always readily available to everyone. It is also immediately gratifying. Sometimes it is not so much entitlement as it is a sense of compensation. They compensate for their perceived underprivileged status by being more willing to spend their money on small luxuries. These small luxuries help them to feel that they are indeed worthy of being pampered. They may spend their money getting tattoos or expensive sneakers, which are viewed as status symbols. Food also gives them this sense of being pampered.

Foods eaten as rewards and entitlements have a very strong tendency to be junk foods, such as candy bars or potato chips. Nobody eats carrot sticks as their reward or entitlement. Doctors and dietitians who suggest substituting celery stalks for candy bars have completely missed the point. The treatment of this problem is discussed in the next chapter under the topic of comfort eating.

I do have a concern regarding treating this attitude of entitlement. As mentioned above, these may sometimes be people who are not really happy with their lives. Food may help to make life bearable by offering some temporary relief from their world. Sometimes the other option would have been escape in the way of alcohol or drugs, which may be worse.

Food as a Surrogate for Love

Another very unhealthy attitude toward food is that food for many people has become a surrogate for many things. Food becomes very entangled with love. This starts out at a very young age when your mother was the one who fed you and the one who loved you. I have noticed a strange phenomenon; whenever we are sick, we tend to want whatever it was our mothers gave us when we were sick as children. My mother used to give me a thin rice porridge when I was ill, so that's what I feel like. My wife used to get liquid Jell-O, so that's what she wants when she is not well. I have a friend who strangely enough always craves hamburgers and fries when he is sick because apparently that's what he got when he did not feel well! Maternal love is not the only kind of love that revolves around food. When we are dating our future or prospective spouses, the dates tend to be around food. In a previous age it used to be told to young women hoping to find a man that, "The way to a man's heart was through his stomach", and young men used to want to find a girl that could "cook like mom!"

While this food-love connection can be quite normal, it becomes unhealthy when it takes the form of comfort eating. These people eat because they are unhappy, lonely, stressed, scared or otherwise in need of comfort. They view food as a surrogate for love.

Food to Make Up For Feelings of Inadequacy

I think that we often use food to cover up our feelings of inadequacy. For example, in today's society where parents hand their children over to day-care, or are too busy and stressed to spend much time with them, parents often let their children get candies, soda pops, as well as expensive toys. If we feel guilty that we are not able to give them as much of ourselves as we feel we should, we do not want to deny them the material things they ask for. Often this ends up being foods high in sugar. This is doubly dangerous because not only do we help make them overweight, we also teach them food as a surrogate for love (see above). There are studies that suggest that obesity rates are higher with permissive parenting styles than with authoritarian parenting styles. Children of divorced families and other single parent families are also at risk.

Gender Differences in Attitudes Toward Food

I suspect that there are real differences in the abnormal attitudes that men and women develop toward food. There is something considered manly or macho about being able to "pack it away". If you were male, you would not want to be accused of eating like a girl. By golly, if you were a *real* man you should order the manly "super-sized" version for only 49 cents more! You even have steakhouses where you can order a 72 oz. Porterhouse that will be free if you can finish it off completely within 2 hours! That is marketed as a feat to prove your masculine prowess, although the only thing I ever considered it to prove was that you were about as dumb as the ox you just consumed!

This masculine pride at being able to overeat is ingrained very deeply in our psyche and our society. Many role models for boys tend to be "Big and Strong", such as professional athletes. We are encouraged to eat to grow up "Big and Strong".

Women on the other hand may overeat for different reasons. For example, women often gain weight following childbirth. Also, in the more traditional family structure, women were more likely to be involved in the preparation of food and be around food all day. This may lead to more all-day grazing.

Socioeconomic Differences in Attitudes Toward Food

We also know that there are differences in the rates of obesity between people of different socioeconomic status as well as between people of different educational attainment. Interestingly, while prosperous nations have more problems with obesity than poorer nations, within the more prosperous nations, obesity is more common among the people of lower socioeconomic status. Education also seems to be protective. In a huge survey of 164,250 people in the year 2000, it was found that African-American women with less than a high school education were *three times as likely* to be morbidly obese as African-American women with four or more years of college education, and *ten times more likely* to be morbidly obese than white men with four or more years of college. These statistics are very important to me because I am far more interested in *why* people overeat rather than *what* they eat.

An interesting finding is that childhood obesity rates are climbing very rapidly in China. One theory advanced is that it is due to the "One Child per Family" policy in China, where it is against the law to have more than one child, except in very exceptional cases. This policy was introduced to curb the rapidly growing population. Could this policy be promoting more permissive parenting and causing the weight gain?

I suspect that most of the differences in obesity rates among different segments of society are related to different unhealthy attitudes toward food. In turn, these lead to the abnormal eating patterns which are responsible for weight gain. Perhaps the most important reason for trying to understand the different socio-cultural roots of obesity is that only by understanding them will we be able to stop the epidemic of obesity, and prevent our children from becoming obese.

> Only by understanding the different socio-cultural roots of obesity will we be able to stop the epidemic of obesity.

The Diet Mentality

A different consequence of these unhealthy attitudes is what I call the "diet mentality". My belief is that if you were to eat like a normal-weight person, in time, your weight will become normal. What I want is for you to normalize your diet and to normalize your attitudes toward food. One of the main underlying abnormal attitudes that overweight people possess is that food is *too* important to them. When they go on a diet, does food become less important to them or more important? People without weight problems do not think of food very often in the day until they get hungry, or until mealtime comes around. Overweight people think too much about food. This is perhaps the *real* abnormality. When they go on a diet, instead of

SIMON FENG, M.D.

thinking less about food, all they can think about is food. Instead of making the problem better, it gets worse! I think that this may be why weight problems keep getting worse with time. Each time a person goes on a diet, food becomes more important. People on diets think about very little else except food all day. I think of dieting as "feeding the problem".

> When people go on a diet, instead of thinking less about food, <u>all they can think about is food</u>. Instead of making the problem better, it gets worse!

Why I Do Not Believe In Calorie Counting or Target Weights

Many patients ask me what their ideal weight should be. You can always look up tables that tell you what your ideal weight is, but I try to discourage this. I believe that it is very difficult to normalize your diet when you are concentrating on things that are unhealthy. Thin people simply do not obsess over what they should weigh and how many calories they should or should not be consuming. The big challenge is to try to get people to think and act like thin people, rather than like fat people trying to lose weight.

> The big challenge is to try to get people to think and act like thin people, rather than like fat people trying to lose weight.

As far as calorie counting is concerned, I do not believe that any diet requiring you to do it has any hope of success because that makes your attitudes toward food more unhealthy instead of less so. I believe the biggest reason that recent popular low-carbohydrate diets have been more successful than many other diets is that they do away with calorie counting. People are able to stay on these diets longer and thus lose more weight.

I will do some calorie counting with you here. I want you to have an idea of how a typical day's calorie balance works, and even here I wish to be deliberately vague. The average person expends somewhere around 1,800 calories a day. Obviously, a 250-pound lumberjack needs more calories than a 125-pound pencil pusher. One pound of fat is roughly worth 3,600 calories, deliberately rounded to be double the average daily caloric requirements (but still fairly accurate), to make the math a lot simpler. This means that if not a single calorie went between your teeth, the fastest you could lose is about ½ pound of fat a day, or 3½ pounds of fat a week. This does not mean that you couldn't lose 10 pounds a week, but at most you would have lost 3½ pounds of fat. You would have lost some muscle and a fair bit of fluid, both of which weigh much more than fat. I would think however that it is really only the fat you wish to lose. If you cut your caloric intake by a little less than 30% you would end up losing one pound a week. Patients always seem to be disappointed by what they perceive to be too slow a rate of weight loss. I wish to point out that this rate is more than 50 pounds in one year as well. It is quite true that the faster you lose weight, the faster it comes back, while the slower the weight loss, the more likely it is to be permanent.

I do wish to point out that not counting calories is not the same as not being aware of what foods are high in calories. I think that it is helpful to know that ranch dressing usually has significantly more calories than Italian dressing, that cheese cake has more calories than a bowl of fresh berries with some whipped cream. People who drink a lot of soda-pop or cappuccinos need to understand the scale of their caloric intake. Even if you are not counting calories, be aware when some choices contain significantly more calories than their alternatives.

> Not counting calories is not the same as not being aware of what foods are high in calories.

Key Differences Between Overweight and Normal Weight People

Dieting strategies are merely ineffective ways to compensate for the abnormal attitudes that cause obesity. The goal of the healing arts should be to return the patient to the normal state if at all possible. The "normal" state is one without abnormal attitudes toward food and the patient can eat normally. None of the treatments available today for obesity seeks to return the patient to this normal condition. Bariatric surgery certainly does not return the patient to the normal state. My hope is that if we can identify the key differences between the overweight people and the normal weight people, we may be able to come up with strategies that truly attempt to return the overweight patient to the normal state! I have not been able to find many studies in the medical literature that looked at behavioral and/or psychological differences between overweight and normal weight people. Some of the differences that have been identified include:

- Overweight people tend to have a lower psychological sense of well-being. It is unclear how much of this is causing weight problems and how much is resulting from being overweight. This is pertinent to the discussion on comfort-eating in the next chapter.
- Overweight people tend to be less physically active.
- Normal weight people eat breakfast more consistently than do overweight people.

> The goal of the healing arts should be to return the patient to the normal state if at all possible. The "normal" state is one without abnormal attitudes toward food and **the patient can eat normally**. None of the treatments available today for obesity seeks to return the patient to this normal condition.

I believe that the biggest differences between people of normal weight and overweight people have never been identified before in the medical literature. These differences are discussed in greater detail in the next chapter as well.

- Overweight people have unhealthy attitudes toward food. Food is too important to them.
- Overweight people have unhealthy eating patterns.

One difference that you will not find is the enjoyment of food. Normal weight people enjoy food every bit as much as their overweight counterparts. I run into people who tell me, "I love food too much to ever lose weight." This is simply and absolutely not true.

> Normal weight people enjoy food every bit as much as their overweight counterparts.

The Sociological Inertia of Culture

A great deal of what I say may seem at first glance to be counter-intuitive and going against normal ways of thinking. People are used to thinking of losing weight by counting calories, using will power, and making a conscious effort to lose weight. As a culture, we like to believe in dogma. We are told what to believe and what is right, and we accept it without having to take the trouble to think it out for ourselves and question if the dogma is correct.

As an example of this phenomenon, consider the following: Many of us will remember breakfast cereal boxes carrying information about the vitamin content of the cereal. This cereal would have 100% of the RDA (recommended daily allowance) of this vitamin and that vitamin, while another brand claimed only to have 80 %. This even led to the "vitamin wars" where cereal companies would fortify their product until it had 100% of the RDA of every water-soluble vitamin.

How many of us stopped to wonder why a two year-old child had the same RDA of Vitamin B1 as a 300-pound NFL linebacker? RDA's were not dependent upon age, sex, weight or level of activity. Who was doing all the "recommendations" anyway? What would happen if you failed to take the RDA of vitamin B6? Why do you have to take your whole day's allotment of vitamins by breakfast in the first place? Well, while none of this was really logical, it sure sold a lot of breakfast cereal!

In my opinion, many of the ways we think about weight loss and dieting belong similarly to illogical patterns of belief entrenched in social inertia and dogma. Let us stop treating abnormalities with more abnormalities when we can achieve a better result by returning to a normal state. We need to stop treating overweight people who have unnatural and unhealthy eating patterns with diets that are still unnatural ways of eating. Instead, we should be helping them to eat normally.

> Let us stop treating abnormalities with more abnormalities when we can achieve a better result by returning to a normal state.

Chapter Seven: Unhealthy Eating Patterns

"To guarantee victory, you need to know yourself
and know your enemy." – Sun Tzu, 5th Century BC China

In the last chapter, I discussed how I believe that the epidemic of obesity has come about largely because we, as a society, have developed some unhealthy attitudes toward food. These unhealthy attitudes then translate into and manifest themselves as unhealthy behaviors involving food, which I categorize into different "Unhealthy Eating Patterns". I believe that the prevention of obesity must lie in finding ways to change our unhealthy attitudes, whereas understanding the Unhealthy Eating Patterns as well can lead us to better treatment of those already afflicted.

> Understanding Unhealthy Attitudes may allow us to prevent obesity.
>
> Understanding Unhealthy Eating Patterns as well may allow us to treat obesity.

I have identified several eating patterns that I feel can lead to weight problems. This list of unhealthy eating patterns may not be complete and other unhealthy patterns may be recognized with time. The patterns discussed here are not mutually exclusive and, more often than not, an overweight person has several patterns that overlap. Also, several different patterns may share some common characteristics. I have separated them into different patterns to make it easier to think about. I deal with some complex issues here that may not be easy to understand the first time you read this. This chapter may well need to be read two or more times.

A very important point that I would like to bring out is that these different unhealthy eating patterns show that different people are overweight for widely different reasons. It is very clear to me that we cannot be treating all our overweight people in the same way if we expect to succeed. This chapter could also have been called "The Different Causes of Obesity".   There are also some other very important differences in different people that have to be taken into account in order to treat their weight problems in a way tailored to the person. These are explored in Chapter Eight.

I believe that these unhealthy eating patterns result in the over-consumption of calories and weight gain. This over-consumption is sometimes unconscious. Correcting the unhealthy eating patterns will result in the desired weight loss.

At the end of this chapter, I have prepared an "Eating Pattern Self-Analysis Chart". The purpose of this chart is to allow you to understand where your abnormal eating patterns are. I think that the treatment each of these categories needs is different. By knowing which categories apply to you and how much it applies to you, you can know what kind of changes you will need to make.

The Unhealthy Patterns

Non-Wasters of Food

This has already been explored in some detail in the last chapter and is a crucial component of my thoughts on permanent weight loss. I believe this to be one of the primary causes of abnormal weight gain. This attitude is so pervasive that we almost all have it to some degree or other. Who among us, for example, hasn't finished a drink or taken a last bite because "it would be a shame not to". We all feel guilty throwing away good food, and especially expensive food.

Money also enters into this abnormal attitude. People in this category often "supersize" their meals because it is a much better a deal, offering so much more food for only a little more money. They think that it would be so much of a waste of money if they got the regular size, then found themselves still hungry and needing to buy more food. Once they buy the food, of course it becomes such a great waste of money if they don't finish it all!

I guess that I need to qualify this a little when I call it an "unhealthy" attitude since it is also almost universal. This attitude is certainly not unhealthy in developing or Third World countries but is now no longer a healthy attitude for us to have in America. It is precisely because we live in the land of plenty, where hunger is rare, that we must work very hard to keep this reluctance to waste food from causing us to gain undesired weight. For most of our history we have had to try to hoard away and store energy for times of famine, but now this trait has become a terrible enemy. Can it be defeated? Yes, of course. Normal weight people do it all the time. They may overeat from time to time but if they overeat at one meal, they will automatically reduce their intake over the next few meals. If a person does not gain any weight over a 10-year period, it does not mean that he or she never once overate. It just means that they would automatically compensate for the over-eating. We all know someone who hasn't gained a pound in ten years. Remember in the last chapter we had gone through some caloric counting? One pound of fat has roughly 3600 calories. Ten years has 3650 days. Therefore, if this person has not gained or lost one pound in that time frame, the calorie intake is balanced to an average of one calorie per day! No dietitian in the world can calculate your diet to that degree of accuracy. I point this out only to illustrate the amazing ability of our bodies to tell us what we need, if we would only learn to listen.

How do we treat this unhealthy pattern? I tell my patients that the first thing they need to do is to totally and completely get rid of their reluctance to waste food. If this is one of the reasons you are overweight, from here on in, throw away food at every meal. Do not ever leave your plate clean. We have to teach your body to once again listen to its signals. We are all born with this ability. Look at how children eat. They only eat until they are no longer hungry. Unfortunately, we teach the children to overeat because we do not let them leave the table until they are forced to eat all their greens or their chicken. We train them to ignore the body's signals to stop eating. If this is how you were taught, it is not really your parent's fault because they were just teaching you the same way that they were taught. Nevertheless, we now have to unlearn decades of conditioning.

From now on, before you begin your meal separate it into 2 halves. After you have eaten the first half, pause for a little to see if you are still hungry. If you are, separate the remaining food into 2 smaller piles and again, pause when you finish the first. If you are really so hungry that you need to finish the whole plate, do so, then get a second helping and push that away. Make sure that you throw away some food at every single meal. I don't care if it is one bite or

SIMON FENG, M.D.

half the plate but make sure you do throw some food away. This may seem really wasteful but it is really important. The idea of this exercise is not necessarily to waste food but to re-train the body's own sense of satiety. You have probably spent many decades training yourself to ignore your body's signal to stop eating; don't be surprised if it takes several months or so to learn when you really should stop. Initially, you may stop eating too soon, or too late, but with time, hopefully you will find your own satiety point because there is no fixed amount of food to be eaten. I will tell you that ***it is much harder to do than it would seem***. You will be surprised the first time you try to throw away a significant amount of food, how ingrained this reluctance to waste food is. It is very hard to throw out good food and it doesn't work if you only throw out the uneaten portion that does not taste that great. Most of us will have little trouble throwing out food that does not need to be eaten if there is only half a bite involved but it is precisely when there is a significant amount left that you really do not need to eat it. It is also really difficult to throw out delicious food or expensive food.

If you find yourself facing food on your plate that you are reluctant to throw away, you must understand that all that food represents extra calories you do not need. This is quite possibly the source of all the calories responsible for you being overweight! In the past, all these calories would have been consumed. If you consider this amount of food to be insignificant, consider this: Overeating by a mere 30 calories per meal will add up to about 10 pounds in one year, and 100 pounds in 10 years! Most of the time it may be quite a bit more than 30 calories per meal you do not need to eat. It should not be a hardship to do without this food because by definition, this is food that you do not need to eat!

If it really bothers you that you are throwing away good food while children are starving in Somalia (even though finishing your plate doesn't help them), this is what I suggest you do. Figure out how much money you spend on food per month. After you have corrected the way you eat, you will find that you are buying less food. Pledge to send that money to UNICEF (United Nations International Children's Emergency Fund) or some other food-aid program. That is how you help the starving children of the world. Can you imagine what an insult it really is to some hungry child in Ethiopia, if she could watch you eat that food saying, "I'm not going to waste this food because you are starving?" The waste lies in *buying* the food in the first place, rather than in not eating it.

If you still feel very strongly that it is immoral to throw good food away, I would strongly suggest that you keep the food as leftovers for the next meal. *The important thing is not to eat it.* Also, the purpose of this exercise of throwing away food is not to waste food but to retrain you to listen to your body.

Learning to leave food uneaten is one of the biggest ways that sets apart how people without weight problems eat from how overweight people eat. Normal weight people can sometimes eat as much as bigger people do, but they only eat that way once in a while. Most of the time, they leave some food uneaten. They stop when they are full.

This problem with not wanting to waste food is not restricted to mealtimes. For example, if you go to a movie and order popcorn, which tastes better - the first inch of popcorn or the last inch? I have never had anyone tell me they preferred the last inch, but my question is then, "Why do you eat the last inch?" The reason the popcorn is finished is because it is there and it would be a waste not to eat it. Also, if we open a can of ice cold cola or beer, by the time you get to the last sip it is no longer as cold or refreshing as the first sip. Still we finish it because it has been paid for. Once the food has been paid for, it doesn't matter anymore whether you eat it or not. The money has been spent. The food either goes to waste or it goes to waist. Never try to get your money's worth.

> Excess food either goes to waste or it goes to waist.
> Never try to get your money's worth.

I wish to emphasize that this treatment of throwing out food or saving food is not the same as portion control. Portion control is really a limitation on temptation, but you will always be tempted to finish the food. There will always be times when you cannot control your portion size, for example, when you are at a restaurant, or at a party with a smorgasbord of food. If you learn to leave food uneaten it will not matter how much food is in front of you. People without weight problems do not practice portion control – they just stop eating when they are full.

SIMON FENG, M.D.

> Portion control is just limiting temptation. Normal weight people do not practice portion control. Learning to stop eating when one is full is the normal, healthy way to eat.

The other effect that finishing the plate has on the way people eat is that while normal weight people eat until they are comfortably full, overweight people do not stop eating until they are uncomfortably full. They learn to interpret this discomfort (feeling "stuffed") as feeling full or satiated, which is also why they tend to overeat. They think that they have larger than normal appetites because they do not feel that they should stop yet when they are only comfortably full. If you always drive ten miles per hour faster than the speed limit, it doesn't feel like you are going fast enough if you're only doing the speed limit. You need to unlearn eating to the point of discomfort. Understand that feeling full is not the same thing as feeling "stuffed".

> Do not mistake feeling "stuffed" for feeling full.
> Unlearn the habit of eating to the point of discomfort.

Food as Entertainment

This group, along with the previous of "non-wasters", represents attitudes that are extremely prevalent, if not universal in our society. Just like the previous category, it has its roots in our past. To my knowledge, there is no culture on earth that does not use food in celebration. The difference here is that whereas in the past (and still today in Third World countries), celebrations and festivals came around infrequently, our culture today can afford to celebrate every day. It has been said that the average person in America today can eat better than any emperor in the past. We can enjoy foods out of season, whether it is grapes in January or ice cream in February. The selection of different foods to tempt our palate is almost inexhaustible. We can have sushi for lunch and prime rib for supper on the same day. Food is also too easy when you can pick up a 3-course dinner in a drive-through.

The easy access to good food and the ability to enjoy feasting on a daily basis can easily lead to using food as a form of entertainment. I enjoy good food as much as the next person, but I feel that we need to understand that this attitude towards food as entertainment can be problematic. Don't panic, I am not advocating that we all go back to eating bland, tasteless food.

While nearly everyone enjoys good food, not everyone is overweight. Why? First of all, I would like to point out that the enjoyment of food is not necessarily associated with the amount of food eaten. Food critics do not have to be obese any more than wine critics need to be alcoholics. It is certainly possible to indulge without overindulging. Most people without weight problems are able to do this. However, the people mentioned in the previous section who always clean off their plates, are chronic overeaters who eat to the point of being uncomfortably full instead of comfortably full. Even though it sounds like a contradiction, these people often enjoy the sensation of being uncomfortably full. They need to unlearn this misinterpretation and enjoy good food for the quality rather than for the quantity.

> Food critics do not have to be obese any more than wine critics need to be alcoholics. It is possible to love food without overindulging.

Celebrate your love for food but never allow yourself to be a slave to food. Food is part of our culture, and indeed most cultures are defined, in part, by their cuisine. It is also part of our social lives. We meet friends over lunch, socialize over supper and serve food at every party. Keep in mind that people without weight problems also enjoy food and have social lives. My whole emphasis in this book has been on normalizing the way we eat. It is normal to enjoy food. At the risk of repeating myself, it is just terribly important to separate the enjoyment of the quality of food from the quantity of food. I, myself, enjoy going to buffets because of the variety of different foods, but I have small portions of different selections. I may have a small second helping of my favorites to savor the taste but I don't eat to the point of discomfort. A word of caution: do not attempt to go to "All-you-can-eat" buffets until you have learned to enjoy food without feeling "stuffed".

> Learn to delight in the quality of food rather than enjoying the quantity of food.

In keeping with my philosophy of normalizing the way we eat, I believe that occasional feasting is normal and allowed. The key is the word "occasional". Allow yourself to over-eat three or four times a year, on special occasions only. It is not the occasional overindulgence that causes the weight problem but the everyday over-consumption. It may be easier to avoid the everyday overeating if you allow yourself the occasional episode on special occasions.

> It is not the occasional overindulgence that causes the weight problem but the everyday over-consumption.

Food is also often used as reward. When we feel that we have had a hard day at work, we may want to reward ourselves with food. Unfortunately, we may have a hard day at work four days a week! I believe this attitude is unhealthy. You can use food as reward for the occasional big achievement such as graduation, a big promotion, or your child winning the state championship in something. You must not use food as a reward for everyday or every week accomplishments. If you need a reward for these, calculate how much money you spend on these "food rewards" and save them up to spend on something you would really like. Food as reward also fits in with comfort eating, discussed below.

I know that this sounds difficult but it really can be done. For those of you who used to smoke and have quit, you will know what I mean. Smokers also use cigarettes as mini-rewards. They use cigarettes as reward after finishing work, after a meeting, after chores are done, after meals and after sex. When they first quit smoking they think about cigarettes after all the above activities, but after a few weeks they can do these activities without automatically thinking about smoking. It is actually easier than it sounds. If we learn to normalize our attitudes towards food, it will be a permanent change.

This category of "Food as Entertainment" can be quite a mixed bag. Therefore, treatments also need to be different. Some people, who are only mildly overweight, recognize the tendency to overindulge and consciously try to curb their eating. As long as they do not lose control and are able to keep fighting their weight to somewhat of a draw, I think it is acceptable, in the absence of other health issues such as diabetes. If they are unhappy with their weight, they should find alternative means of entertainment.

Unfortunately, there are also those who become very overweight with their unbridled enjoyment of food. My suspicion is that there are self-esteem issues for many of these people. After battling the world all day, they may return home at night and find that food is the only enjoyment they really have. They may have limited social skills that could give them alternative types of entertainment. This group overlaps with the "comfort eating" group discussed later in this chapter. Their psychological problems need to be addressed, and they probably would benefit from learning other coping mechanisms. Anti-depressants and psychotherapy may be beneficial. These patients need to divorce food from self-esteem. They are often slaves to their food and they need to declare their independence.

A subgroup of this category of food for entertainment includes males for whom overindulgence was considered as a desirable "macho" trait. As children, their parents would be proud of how much food they could eat. When they go to a buffet they will proudly display their manly prowess by demonstrating how much they can eat. This is an extremely important category to recognize, especially for those of us with male children, that we do not encourage this dangerous association.

> Please! Do not encourage "Macho" eating in children.

As mentioned at the start of this section, the use of food as entertainment is universal. Quite often, other abnormal eating patterns may co-exist. I strongly suggest that other unhealthy eating patterns be looked for.

Avoidance of Public Eating / Meal Skippers

One very important feature of the way many overweight people eat is that how you see them eat in public is often only the very tip of the iceberg. Even if you feel you know them very well, perhaps working beside them for many years, you never see them eat when they are alone. Overweight people tend to have a real aversion to eating in public. I think that this is understandable. They feel that if they are seen eating a large amount of food, other people will think, "No wonder that person is so fat!" On the other hand, people seeing them eating only a little will think, "Boy, I'm surprised how little that big person eats. It must be their metabolism!"

> Overweight people tend to have a real aversion to eating in public.

However, this type of eating behavior often leads to some very undesirable effects. Often, these people feel hungry a few hours later and snack on candy bars or potato chips, or something else with empty calories. They feel that they can justify this, seeing how little they had eaten earlier. They end up consuming far more calories than a decent meal would have given them.

It is also very commonly with this group that they skip breakfast, because this is the easiest meal to skip. All you have to do is sleep in an extra 15 minutes and you don't have time for breakfast. Lunch at work is usually eaten in front of your colleagues and co-workers, so it is easy to eat little if anything for lunch. Now when they get home, they are really starving. They feel that they have been good all day so they should be entitled to eat. They often spend the rest of the evening constantly eating and grazing until they have put away phenomenal amounts of food, not uncommonly in excess of 2,000 calories at one sitting. (This may overlap with the Binge Eater described later in this chapter.) Meanwhile, during the day they may have already consumed 750 to 1,000 calories in sodas or iced teas. In the worst form, these patients may become bulimic, making themselves vomit up all the food that they have already eaten.

The other very important thing that happens to meal skippers is that they may actually consume more calories from snacking and drinking throughout the day than they would have, had they had a normal breakfast and lunch. These calories are also more likely to be empty calories, high in carbohydrates, low in proteins, vitamins and minerals as well as fiber. This kind of diet also may cause your body to break down muscle mass and lean body mass to get proteins and amino acids that are missing in the diet. The end result of this is that while you may be gaining weight you are actually suffering from malnutrition.

The treatment for this type of eating abnormality is obvious. Start eating three proper meals a day. If you have a decent breakfast, you really ought not to be getting hungry until lunchtime, and similarly a proper lunch should hold you till supper. Many people feel that it is impossible to eat three meals a day and not gain weight. They seem to be convinced that this will cause their weight to balloon up. If that is how you think, it should be a real sign of how far you have departed from a normal diet and thinking normally about food. Just remember that people without weight problems almost always eat this way! Most overweight people do not really have an unhealthy metabolism, just an unhealthy attitude, and a resultant unhealthy diet. The only people who deliberately miss meals and won't eat in public are fat people trying to lose weight. Stop eating like them and start eating like normal people.

> Most overweight people do not really have an unhealthy metabolism, just an unhealthy attitude.

I would like to point out that this type of unhealthy eating pattern usually represents a secondary form of abnormality. Primary abnormalities represent those which made the person overweight in the first place, whereas secondary abnormalities are unhealthy eating patterns that developed after the person became overweight. Because these abnormalities may be secondary, one needs to identify other unhealthy eating pattern(s) that may exist and correct them as well.

This aversion that many overweight people have to eating in public may contribute to the commonly held notion that the overweight condition is caused by genetic/metabolic problems. Because we do not see our overweight co-workers and friends eating a lot of food, it is so much easier and kinder to assume overweight people suffer from an unfortunate metabolism.

The Grazer

This form of unhealthy eating pattern is also fairly common. I believe that this can be either a primary abnormality or a secondary one. The person who practices this kind of eating behavior is constantly eating throughout the day. He or she usually does not have any idea of how many calories are consumed, although sometimes the person just does not care.

If they truly do not care, there is very little that we can do for them except to point out the potential or actual harm that they may be inflicting upon themselves. Often these individuals are teenagers who do not fit well with the "popular" crowd at school and as teenagers they do not see the future consequences of their behavior. Teenagers also tend to see things as all black or all white, and once they give up on their appearance, they really do not care.

The treatment for this group is quite simple on the surface: stop all the snacks and eat only at mealtimes. However, as may be seen from the above discussion, there may well be other psychological factors that may need to be addressed, such as teenage depression.

The secondary form of this kind of eating pattern is represented by people who were overweight to begin with. They are very conscious of overeating at mealtimes and get hungry between meals and end up snacking. At the next meal they feel guilty for their previous snacking and so eat only a little. This sets up the vicious cycle where they find themselves hungry again a short while later and feel they can justify a little snack because they really did not eat much at lunch. Of course, suppertime finds them feeling guilty again and the pattern repeats all the way to bedtime.

The secondary form of this abnormal eating pattern is very similar to the meal skipper. The biggest differences are that these people are not self-conscious about eating in public, and they eat small meals rather than skipping meals. The reason that they do not each much at mealtime is motivated by fear of calories, rather than being self-conscious about eating in public. There may also be overlap with "liquid calories" (described later in this chapter), as grazers tend to consume a lot of beverages that may contain a lot of unrecognized calories.

One big problem with this pattern of eating is that the foods that form the snacks are usually high calorie junk food, from doughnuts to cookies to candy or chocolates. These calories add up very fast. These may also be the people who honestly think that they really don't eat much and must be overweight because of some abnormal metabolism. They are unaware of the calories they have actually consumed.

The treatment for this group is, once again, to correct the abnormal eating patterns. Eat your regular meals and you really should not be getting hungry until close to the next mealtime. Make sure that any underlying psychological issues are dealt with. Psychotherapy and/or medication may be necessary.

The Sweet Tooth

Sugar is immediately available energy. It is the most basic fuel at the cellular level. No wonder it has such appeal. If you offered any laboratory animal sugared water and regular water at the same time, it will almost always go for the sweetened water. Similarly, given a choice between regular breakfast cereal and sweetened cereal, kids will pick the latter every time.

This has not been a big problem historically. If you went back a hundred years ago, refined sugar was just not that readily available. Again, throughout many diverse and different cultures, special treats for children tend to be sweet. It was just never this readily available till the past 50 years. Sugar was always associated with joy, comfort, and reward. The problem is that as our society has prospered, we can now afford these special treats all the time. Cakes and cookies and candies that used to be served only at festivals and holidays are now available year-round. No longer are they only to be found around Christmas and birthdays. Kids now feel deprived if they don't have a cookie or other sweet treat in their lunch box. Soft drinks are now also a staple. It has only been in the last 30 years or so that kids could buy any kind of treat they wished out of a vending machine at school.

This association of sugar and joy/love/reward persists easily into adulthood. What do we give our kids at Easter or Halloween but candy? We call our romantic partners "sweethearts" and woo them with chocolates on Valentine's Day. If you are older and you have grandchildren coming over, better get busy in the kitchen cooking up all those goodies!

My solution? Well, it may too late for some people to dissociate sugar from all those warm and fuzzy feelings. We need to re-examine the messages we are giving our children. We need to limit

SIMON FENG, M.D.

the sugar they get. I had a patient who told me, "But Doctor, he won't drink plain water!" My response was, 'Of course not, when he is rewarded with soda-pop if he holds out long enough!" One problem is that overweight parents remember (perhaps unconsciously) all the warm and fuzzy feelings they had when they received sweets as children. They do not wish to deprive their children of these wonderful feelings. I think sweet treats are fine but they just need to be limited. Allow the kids to come home with their Halloween loot, but three days later, chuck all the candy out. There is no need to be celebrating Halloween for the next three weeks.

> Occasional sweet treats are fine but need to be limited. Throw out all remaining candy three days after Halloween. There is no reason to celebrate Halloween for the next three weeks.

For the adults who already have been hurt by their sweet tooth, make a conscious effort to limit it to no more than once a week. If you really feel the need to eat a candy bar, buy one, take no more than two bites then throw the rest away (See above discussion on reluctance to "waste" food). If you have to partake of something sweet, select products that use sugar alternatives such as NutraSweet® or Splenda®. Often you need time to adjust to the different taste of the sugar substitute, but in time they will not taste bad at all.

It is not that I am such a big advocate of putting synthetic chemicals, such as sugar substitutes, into your body, but I think that for the weight-conscious it may be the lesser of evils. I would far rather you just drink water in place of diet pop, but I also realize that sometimes that may not be realistic.

Liquid Calories

For some, the majority of their calories comes from drinking sweetened drinks, whether we are talking about sodas or Kool-Aid or sweetened tea. The caloric intake can be very high indeed. I have known many a patient who consumed an average of ten cans of soda per day. Many people do not realize how much sugar there is in a can of soda (12oz). Believe it or not, there are about 10 teaspoons of sugar in a single can. If you were to watch me put 10 teaspoons of sugar in my coffee you would blink disbelievingly and probably gag. At an average of 150 calories per can, this adds up very quickly to 1,500 calories, which is almost the entire day's requirement. All this before the poor person has even eaten one bite! It has gotten even worse, as there is a definite trend for portion sizes to increase in recent years. Now I see many people with 20-oz pop bottles, which of course have about 250 calories in each bottle. Liquid calories are not restricted to soda pops. Fruit juices also contain a similar amount of sugar. For example, orange juice contains about 120 calories per 8 ounce serving, which is almost as high as soda. The new trendy café lattes and cappuccinos are also very high in calories, being high in fat as well as sugar. Sugared ice teas are not much better.

Clearly, people in this category need to stop or seriously curtail their sugar intake. The ideal solution is to switch to water, and to this end I am happy to see people toting around bottles of spring water. I have never figured out why water costs so much but I think bottled water is a truly wonderful trend which has made it so much more acceptable to be drinking water instead of something with calories. I would like to see all the people in this category switch to water, but that is not always realistic, at least in the short term. We also need to be very careful about their caffeine intake, which is typically very high in many types of sodas. If these people switched over to water in one swoop they would likely be incapacitated with headaches. I typically ask them to switch to diet soda and alternate with a caffeine-free diet drink (such as alternating diet coke with caffeine-free diet coke or diet sprite and gradually replacing these with water, if possible).

Almost all these patients tell me they hate the taste of diet sodas. What I tell them is that almost always they will get used to it. Most of us now drink 1%, 2% or skim milk, but if you think back to when you first switched over from whole milk, 2% milk didn't even taste like "real" milk. However, if you were to try whole milk now, you would feel like you were drinking straight cream. In other words, once you get used to it after a few weeks, you won't mind the diet taste anymore. In fact, a lot of people end up telling me they prefer the taste of diet soda to regular soda. Ask any person who drinks diet sodas and they will confirm this. The same is true of people who salt their food heavily. Initially they feel that there is no taste to their food, but once they are used to it, they can't go back to all that salt.

SIMON FENG, M.D.

It is crucial that when these people go off their sweetened drinks, they do not replace the drinks with other sweet treats. If they lose all their drinks without otherwise changing anything, they should lose a significant amount of weight.

A note of caution: Some people who drink this much may have diabetes, which can make them very thirsty. Get checked.

A special case of the liquid calorie person is the alcoholic. Obviously, treatment of these people is beyond the scope of this book.

Comfort Eating

This is a very common phenomenon and can take very different forms in different people. It can range in severity from mild to very severe. It can occur as a primary eating abnormality that causes weight problems, but sometimes it is a secondary form that complicates other forms of unhealthy eating patterns.

I believe that it starts out because of the very close relationship between nourishment and nurturing. For many people, love equals food, food equals comfort, and food represents safety and freedom from want. We hear it said that chocolate contains a chemical that stimulates the brain the same way that love does. While the object of your desires may reject you, you are always safe with food. If you try to think the way people thought a hundred years ago or so, you will realize that to have food meant you were safe from hunger and famine. It brings to mind the picture of Scarlet O'Hara in "Gone with the Wind" shaking her fists in the air and proclaiming, "As God is my witness, I shall never go hungry again!" Food is such a powerful synonym for comfort and safety that it is not hard to understand why so many reach for food when they are in need of solace.

Sometimes the comfort eating is severe indeed. I remember one patient of mine who had been the victim of repeated incestuous molestation as a child by more than one family member. She had a history of quite a few failed relationships. She had been slender and quite attractive but was so uncomfortable under her own skin that she sought to put on an armor of fat. She felt that if she were fat, only someone who loved her for herself and recognized her inner beauty would want her. She gained a great deal of weight. She eventually got to the point that she needed to lose weight. There was obviously a multitude of psychological issues at play here. There was a lot of unhappiness and comfort eating, some self-loathing, poor self-esteem, a sense of betrayal, and because of the incestuous molestation history, even a fear of intimacy and comfort. In many ways she felt that it was going to be impossible for her to find happiness. Yet, she was not clinically depressed. I told her that she would definitely benefit from psychotherapy. I wasn't sure if psychotherapy could ever get her to where we would really have a good chance of permanent weight loss. She also had a bad family history of heart disease so when she requested bariatric surgery, I was not at all opposed. I do not think that it is reasonable to believe that every case of unhealthy eating will respond to behavioral or attitude changes, and there is definitely a place for bariatric surgery.

Fortunately, not every case of comfort eating is that severe. With comfort eating, the treatment is often a "chicken or egg" thing. A lot of the poor self-esteem and comfort-eating behavior is secondary to the fact that one is overweight. The excess weight may have been gained through comfort eating while going through a rough time with divorce, unemployment or other similar stress, but once there, it perpetuates itself. Comfort eaters are overweight because they are unhappy, but they are also unhappy because they are overweight.

The other huge reason for comfort eating is the unhealthy attitude of viewing food as a reward or entitlement, as previously described. This is such an important phenomenon that I feel it bears repeating. Basically, many people are not happy with their lives and get little or no joy out of day-to-day living. They want or need something that can make themselves feel good. They feel that they are entitled to some form of joy to make life bearable, or they use food to compensate for an unsatisfactory life. This enjoyment often comes in the way of food because it is readily available and provides immediate gratification. After a hard day at work, and by the time the kids are finally in bed, there is little choice of enjoyment except food and TV. Oh, what a deadly combination that makes!

Comfort eating as a manifestation of using food as reward also frequently involves the consumption of sweet foods or junk food. It is very important to find some other form of reward that is more appropriate. As mentioned previously in the book, this eating out of a sense of entitlement allows the overweight person to rationalize inappropriate eating (which they even recognize as inappropriate) by telling themselves that "I deserve it!" It is important to learn to stop rationalizing away the harmful nature of comfort eating. What this kind of rationalization really represents is, knowing that you are lying to yourself, but choosing to believe your own lies anyways.

While not really a form of comfort eating, sometimes eating food out of a sense of entitlement comes after exercise. After working out for 2 hours on the tennis courts, sometimes people feel they deserve to eat and end up overeating by a great deal.

The treatment of comfort eating is first and foremost to recognize the behavior. All underlying depression must be treated, whether by medication, psychotherapy or both. Psychotherapy may be of great help but is not always readily available. Often, it is not really a clinical depression but just unhappiness or dissatisfaction with one's life choices. It can also be very important to find some alternate methods of stress-management or stress-reduction, such as an exercise program, meditation or picking up a new hobby.

I believe very strongly that the best treatment for this kind of problem is not deprivation, in the way of not allowing you to eat what you wish, but replacement. Comfort eaters are using food to substitute for something in their lives; proper treatment entails identifying whatever this something is, and replacing the food with something more appropriate.

> I believe very strongly that the best treatment for this kind of problem is not deprivation but replacement.

Try to identify the source(s) of your unhappiness. If you are a lonely widow who lives alone without much social interaction, you need to get some kind of social life. Join a club; volunteer your services, whether at a hospital or a soup-line. I am not even talking about trying to find a new mate but just get out there and find a reason to get enthusiastic about life again. Sometimes people are reluctant to get a social life because they feel "fat" and they do not feel that the "fat" person is who they really are. They would rather lose weight and then go out, but it may well work much better the other way. They may find it much easier to lose weight if they were to have a social life. Remember the "chicken or egg" thing.

What other rewards can you give yourself? I often ask my patients to think of the time when they will be retired. What would they like to do that they have never had time to do? Everybody has a dream. They may be too embarrassed to tell me their dream when I ask them, but I know everyone has a dream. Maybe it is to write a book or to learn to play a musical instrument. Well, go out and buy that guitar you always wanted to learn to play. Reward yourself with your dream rather than with food. Perhaps you wanted to get a college degree. Imagine working on your degree by correspondence courses. Two years later, you have the degree you've always wanted and lost 50 pounds in the process. How much better could it get?

I feel it is important to give more possible examples because comfort eaters need to see that it is possible to find some other passion beside food. At the risk of going on a little too much with examples, I knew someone who put together a sports car from spare pieces he found on the internet. I had a patient who lost a lot of weight starting up a new business at home at night, becoming a bladesmith making special-order knives. Now, he travels to many trade shows in several states and makes a good living from his "hobby". If you tend to do all your comfort eating at night (a very common pattern), it is not enough just to have a day-time hobby but you must have a passion that involves working on it in the evenings.

> If you tend to do all your comfort eating at night (a very common pattern), it is not enough just to have a day-time hobby but you must have a passion that involves working on it in the evenings.

Other possibilities: research your genealogy on the internet, find a long-lost friend or relative, or write poetry. The possibilities are endless. Everybody has a dream. You may not even remember your own dream but I know you have one. Whatever it is, find it and get started on your dream!

SIMON FENG, M.D.

Binge Eating

Most of us like ice cream, but we don't eat a tubful of it in one sitting. People who binge eat can polish off a whole box of chocolates, a whole bag of cookies or even a whole jar of peanut butter in one sitting. This is obviously a very unhealthy way to eat. These binges usually happen after something stressful has occurred. Whether the boss yelled at them at work, or some interpersonal relationship has gone sour, these people turn to food for comfort and company. Usually the food selected is high in sugar, and there is considerable overlap with the sweet tooth as well as comfort eating. Often there is a sense of abandoning reason or caution. There is an "I don't care if I get fat!" attitude. There may be an unconscious attempt at self-punishment for a perceived failure. The punishment for this perceived failure is obesity, which feels like it is deserved. Following the binge, there is usually immense guilt. There is also the sense of hopelessness in that the patient knew that he or she was doing something they shouldn't be doing but felt powerless to stop it. The combination of guilt and powerlessness is particularly destructive to one's sense of self-esteem. In the worst cases it may deteriorate into bulimia or anorexia nervosa, which are beyond the scope of this book.

It can be somewhat like a food addiction, the way alcoholics turn to alcohol when they feel unable to cope with pressures. They know that they shouldn't but cannot help it. There is no use in telling bingers that they shouldn't binge – they already know this.

It is easy to see this vicious cycle of poor self-esteem causing self-destructive behavior, in turn causing guilt and even worsening self-esteem. How does one get out of this spiral? I can only tell you how I view food addictions. Having been in medical practice for almost 20 years, I noticed that I have never met a binge eater who was happy. Their bingeing may be a form of self-punishment. They do not like themselves. Conversely, every recovered binger got better only when they told themselves, "I deserve better than this!" Even more than that, they told themselves, "I deserve to be happy!"

Binge eating is of course very similar to comfort eating, as they both stem from the same or similar causes. Treatment would be very similar. Especially important may be psychotherapy.

Dieting

Yes, I do consider dieting to be an unhealthy eating pattern. It is in fact one of the most common unhealthy patterns in the obese and possibly one of the most destructive. It accentuates many of the other abnormal eating patterns. For example, meal-skipping may begin as an attempt to diet. The relationship between dieting and binging is also very strong. Usually, one of the main underlying problems in overweight people is that they think too much about food, and food is far too important. For dieters, thoughts about food become all consuming. If normal people use food as entertainment, food can become the dieter's favorite form of entertainment and even, possibly, their obsession.

Why do I say that dieting is possibly one of the most destructive unhealthy eating patterns? I believe without the slightest doubt that dieting greatly reinforces the abnormal ways we think about food and the abnormal attitudes we have toward food. The success rate of diets in long-term weight loss is not good. This of course knocks down our self-esteem when we try our hardest and "fail". We are demoralized. When we feel defeated, where do we turn for solace? Too often the answer is... *food*! The vicious cycle of poor self-esteem leading to comfort eating, causing weight gain, which in turn further degrades self-esteem is greatly accentuated by dieting.

Another example of the destructive nature of dieting can be found in yo-yo dieting. There is no disagreement among weight loss professionals that this is not good for your body or your psyche.

People on diets stand in front of mirrors a great deal, inspecting their own bodily imperfections. Again, an unhealthy self body-image sets in and triggers the vicious cycle of poor self-esteem and comfort eating. I cannot count how many times I have seen young women (in particular) who are not in the least overweight go on diets in search of an ideal magazine-cover body. Years later, they end up overweight, in my opinion because they have induced unhealthy attitudes and eating patterns they might not otherwise have had. There is also evidence from several studies showing that efforts by parents to control and limit their children's eating behavior have the opposite effect of putting their children at greater risk of obesity.

SIMON FENG, M.D.

I would like to draw a curious connection between what I say about dieting and low-carbohydrate diets. I have mentioned before that low-carbohydrate diets seem to enjoy more success than most other diets in terms of amount of weight lost and length of time of weight loss maintenance. I believe that the relative success of these diets is due to the fact that you do not count calories and you eliminate sweets (and in so doing, eliminate snacking). Indirectly, this leads to 3 meals a day and no snacks and no dieting mentality. This is as close to a "Normal Eating Pattern" as you can find in most weight loss programs. This, I believe is the real reason for the relative success of low-carbohydrate diets. One of the main theories that I put forward in this book is that if you lose your "Unhealthy Eating Pattern(s)" and develop a "Normal Eating Pattern", you will lose weight permanently and healthily. The problem with low-carbohydrate diets, as I see it, is that by eliminating carbohydrates, which is the favorite food for many, it still breeds a dieting mentality. People on these diets are still depriving themselves of food they love, and as the adage goes, "Absence makes the heart grow fonder!" Eventually, they still think about their favorite foods too much. It is still not a "normal" way of eating. These people still do not learn to deal with not wasting food, eating for entertainment, or any of the other forms of unhealthy attitudes or eating patterns.

The dieting mentality is not always easy to shake. There are people on perpetual diets and other people who are essentially addicted to being on a diet.

Eating out of Boredom/ Eating to Stay Awake

The prototype of this abnormal form of eating is possibly the commuter. Spending endless hours on the road in traffic often leads to snacking in the car. Sometimes there is a tendency to get drowsy in the car, and eating might be helpful in trying to stay awake. Sometimes it is just boredom. The important thing to realize is that food consumed in these circumstances is not for nourishment, not for enjoyment and not for comfort. It is just to pass the time.

Other things you can do to pass the time should be instituted. One of the simplest alternatives is sugar-free chewing gum or bubble-gum. You can also sing along with the radio. Books on cassettes are available at many libraries and they are wonderful ways to pass the time in the car. I would really prefer that you do not eat while driving as this has been shown to be unsafe. People eating in the car may not be paying enough attention to the road or keeping both hands on the steering wheel. If you do not eat in the car, please do not start this bad habit.

If you are someone who drives for a living or commutes long distances and find it impossible to give up eating in the car, you need to prepare some low calorie snacks, such as carrot sticks, which you can nibble away a bit at a time. To pass the time, count in your head the number of times you chew each bite of carrot and make a game out of how many times you can chew before you have to swallow. The goal is to pass the time. While I stated earlier that it is not feasible to replace reward foods with celery sticks, this is different because this type of snacking is not done for enjoyment or reward but just to pass the time. Other food items to consider may include a bag of grapes or some sunflower seeds in the husks. Chewing gum is a good alternative.

If you eat in the car in order to stay awake, I would strongly recommend that you try to get more sleep and exercise. Consider car-pooling to have somebody to talk to.

If you are eating out of boredom in a setting other than in a car, you have other options. Read a novel or listen to music. Cross-word puzzles are good time-passers.

SIMON FENG, M.D.

How We Become Overweight

I have listed above, the different types of eating patterns that end up causing an over-consumption of calories. I wish to discuss how these unhealthy eating patterns may interact with each other and where the unhealthy attitudes come in. There are basically two different paths to overeating: *Too Many Calories at Mealtimes* and *Too Many Calories between Meals*.

The aversion to wasting food plays a very central role in over-eating at mealtimes. This aversion when combined with factors such as the fixed portion size ("quantumization of food") necessarily leads to overeating! If you are served more food than you need but cannot stop eating until your plate is clean, how can you avoid overeating? Serving smaller portions often leads to hunger between meals and from there to snacking and "too many calories between meals". This is, of course, the other path to overeating.

Similarly, the aversion to wasting food in the context of using food as entertainment, explains why overweight people eat to the point of discomfort rather than just eating to the point of comfort. The better the food, the more of a shame it is not to finish it; therefore, eating to the point of discomfort becomes strongly entrenched in the enjoyment of good food. This is why the enjoyment of food too often becomes the enjoyment of quantity instead of quality. These are some of the reasons why it is so important to lose this aversion to wasting food, or never developing it in the first place for our children.

People who eat too many calories between meals can fall into two categories: those with *Unhealthy Attitudes* and those with *Underlying Psychological Issues*.

The unhealthy attitudes of using food as rewards or entitlements as well as the enjoyment of quantity over quality all play a role. Normal weight people also enjoy snacks but just not in the same order of magnitude as some overweight people. People without weight problems may enjoy ice cream occasionally but some overweight people eat ice cream on a regular basis. Also, instead of one scoop, it is three. Underlying psychological issues need to be dealt with.

Do not be frustrated if you are not sure which of these categories apply to you. They are not mutually exclusive and it is absolutely possible to overeat at mealtimes as well as between meals, have unhealthy attitudes and also underlying psychological issues.

Natural Weight Loss Through Normal Eating

If there is one radical idea in this book, this is it: It is possible to lose weight eating in a totally normal manner. I have tried to introduce this idea gradually by discussing different unhealthy eating patterns and showing how we might be able to correct the abnormal eating pattern and develop a more normal one. Overweight people are scared to bits of eating normally. They are too used to the idea that they must diet and deprive themselves of food in order to lose weight. There is this "No pain, no gain" concept that for a diet to work, you must fight with your cravings and deprive yourself.

> If there is one radical idea in this book, this is it: ***It is possible to lose weight eating in a totally normal manner!***

Many overweight people, especially the meal skippers, cannot believe that you can eat three meals and lose weight because they only eat one meal a day and still gain weight. They don't take account of the fact that they are either snacking during the day, or they eat more calories in their one meal a day than other people do in three meals.

People also do not believe that you can enjoy what you eat and lose weight. Enjoyment of food is all related to the quality of the food, not to the amount of food eaten. If you have trouble believing this, ask yourself this, "Would you enjoy one slice of your favorite dessert more or one pound of carrot sticks more?" Ask any person who is not overweight if they enjoy their food and they will reassure you that they do. It is definitely possible to enjoy your food without overeating.

> It is definitely possible to enjoy your food without overeating.

SIMON FENG, M.D.

What Then Is Normal?

This is not an unreasonable question as I believe that most overweight people no longer have any idea of what normal is. The simplest way is to define Normal as "What", "How" and "Why" normal weight people eat.

<u>What Normal Weight People Eat</u>
Obviously, as a physician, I would much prefer that you make smart choices and eat low fat food with lots of fiber and with adequate variety to ensure a well balanced diet. However, in the absence of medical reasons such as diabetes, high cholesterol or gluten- enteropathy, I will only recommend that you have a healthy diet. Because I believe that it is very important that people enjoy their food, I do not like to prohibit any kind of food. People without weight problems do not really have any restrictions on the type of food that they eat, and I feel this is also not unrealistic for people wishing to lose weight.

I do however believe in moderation. You really cannot be drinking five or six sodas a day if you do not want to be overweight. Sugar needs to be limited, not used as a reward and not used as a surrogate for emotional fulfillment. Excess fat also needs to be avoided. We have mentioned carbohydrates several times but do not forget that fat in the diet is also a big problem for anyone wishing to lose weight. Apart from weight issues, fat in foods contribute to heart disease. Do not count calories but be aware of what foods are high in calories. Be mindful of what you eat.

<u>How Normal Weight People Eat</u>
People without weight problems stop eating when they are no longer hungry. They eat to the point of being comfortably full while overweight people eat to the point of being uncomfortably full.

As mentioned earlier, feasting is a phenomenon that spans across all cultures. Part of the reason for the epidemic of obesity, I think, is that we are now able to feast every day. It is really not the occasional overeating that causes serious weight gain but the everyday overeating. An occasional ice cream is fine but it should not be a triple scoop and it should not be a daily event. Enjoy food for the quality rather than the quantity.

Normal weight people do not miss meals on a regular basis. They do not avoid eating in public. They do not binge. They do not go on diets!

Why Normal Weight People Eat

Many overweight people eat for all the wrong reasons. Normal weight people do not eat because they are stressed or unhappy. They do not use food as a reward or as their refuge from reality. Their lives do not revolve around food. In other words, normal weight people do not have *unhealthy attitudes toward food*, which is one of the main ideas of this book!

How To Deal With Hunger

I often use the model of thirst to deal with hunger. When you are thirsty, it is usually not a catastrophe: you get something to drink. However, you do not hide in a closet to drink, you don't have to drink a whole two liter bottle of soda just because you've opened it and it doesn't have to be soda. Conversely, if you are not thirsty and someone offers you a drink, you don't have to accept it.

Hunger should be treated in the same way. It is normal to feel a little hungry especially around mealtimes. Normal weight people get hungry at times. Just treat it like thirst. If you get hungry and the next meal isn't for a while, get a small snack but just enough to tide you over till the next meal. The idea is to take the edge off, not to fill up. Perhaps an apple or banana would be a good choice. A small slice of cheese or a small serving of low-fat yogurt can also be appropriate.

To summarize, the key to permanent weight loss is to eat normally. This involves the following:

1. Eating three good meals a day: breakfast, lunch and dinner. My preference as a physician is of course that the meal be not too high in fat and not excessive in carbohydrates either. It is important that you enjoy your food.
2. Learning not to overeat at meals by getting rid of your aversion to wasting food and by learning to enjoy the quality of food instead of the quantity. Learn to enjoy the sensation of being comfortably full instead of being uncomfortably full.

SIMON FENG, M.D.

> 3. While it is permissible to snack, until you have normalized your attitudes toward food, limit snacks only to the times when you are actually hungry and the next mealtime is not for some time. Do not snack because you deserve a reward – go find some other more appropriate reward. Do not snack because you are bored or unhappy – find more appropriate replacements for food.

Understand and correct any unhealthy attitudes toward food and deal with any underlying psychological issues involving food.

KEYS TO EATING NORMALLY
1. Enjoy 3 good meals a day.
2. Learn not to overeat at mealtimes.
3. Minimize snacking.

Eating Patterns Self-Analysis Chart

The other really important point that I have tried to show is that different people become overweight through very different unhealthy eating patterns. How can we treat them all the same way? The person who is overweight from drinking too much soda cannot respond to the same treatment plan as the person who skips meals. In order to normalize your eating habits we must identify what you are doing wrong.

I have described the different ways in which people's eating patterns can get them in trouble. It is now time to figure out how many and which of these patterns describe how you eat. To facilitate this, I have listed all the described patterns in table form at the end of this section. This table is entitled, Eating Patterns Self-Analysis Chart.

Beside the unhealthy eating pattern is a column labeled "Severity Category". Mark down a "0" if you do not feel that this eating pattern is part of your problem, a "1" if you think it is a mild problem, "2" if it is moderate and "3" if you think that this is your main problem. Do not be upset if you mark down several categories as number 3, as this is certainly possible. Also do not be upset if you end up marking almost every category.

FENG'S WAY: TO PERMANENT WEIGHT LOSS

Once you have identified the abnormal patterns of how you eat, the last column on the right lists some of the recommended actions you need to consider. Please go back and re-read the sections pertaining to your type of eating pattern(s) until you understand them well. Tackle the 3's and 2's before the 1's.

A word of caution: sometimes when you try to make a change in one category, another abnormal pattern of eating may develop. Also, sometimes old habits come back. If you are having trouble losing weight, you may need to re-evaluate and re-analyze your eating patterns from time to time. For this reason, I prepared an extra copy of the Self-Analysis Charts to use at a later time.

There is a very important concept that does not come across well in the Self-Analysis Chart. It is very important to understand that what I wish is not that you just change the way you eat but also change the way you think about food. Rather than just to deprive yourself of sodas, I want you to lose the association between sugar and thirst. Learn to enjoy quality of food rather than quantity. Learn that it is not sinful to leave food uneaten. These are not easy habits to break and you may need time for new habits to form. You have spent decades learning to eat for the wrong reasons. Give yourself several months to unlearn these old habits and learn some new healthy ones.

> You have spent decades learning to eat for the wrong reasons. Give yourself several months to unlearn these old habits and learn some new healthy ones.

I also want you to understand that I am not talking about depriving yourself of what you want. Instead I wish you to find ways to replace what you want with something you would like even more. For example, if you eat late at night to reward yourself for a hard day's work, I am not suggesting that you do not reward yourself. I am suggesting that you reward yourself with something other than sitting yourself in front of a television set with a bowl of chips. After all, this kind of mindless eating is not all that rewarding. What you really want is a reward but not necessarily a reward in the form of food. Find a more meaningful reward.

Similarly, if your main problem is one of being unable to leave food uneaten, you should not feel it to be a form of deprivation to not eat it. By definition, this food is food that you do not need.

The Eating Patterns Self-Analysis Chart is only to help simplify and organize how you think about your unhealthy eating patterns. There is much information in the body of this chapter and the previous one which could not be included in the chart but needs to be understood to deal effectively with the unhealthy patterns. It is not sufficient to just understand the unhealthy eating patterns but it is also crucial to understand the underlying unhealthy attitudes as well (which were responsible for the unhealthy eating patterns in the first place). I would again encourage you to re-read the chapter on unhealthy attitudes. You may need to jot down the key points on a separate sheet of paper to remind yourself of any information that applies specifically to you.

Let me explain what I mean in a different way: Many people will focus on this chart as the main message or meat of my book, but that is only partially correct. Most weight loss programs in the past have concentrated on <u>what you eat</u>. This Eating Patterns Self-Analysis Chart helps you to focus on <u>how you eat</u>. The Unhealthy Attitudes address <u>why you eat</u>. The extreme importance of how you eat may be lost if you focus only on the chart.

EATING PATTERNS SELF-ANALYSIS CHART (Initial)

Date Completed:

Unhealthy Eating Pattern	Severity Category 0	1	2	3	Suggested Action
Non-Waster of Food					Leave food uneaten at every meal. Do not equate food with money.
Food as Entertainment					Enjoy **quality** of food, not **quantity**. Find alternate forms of reward. Avoid "Macho" eating.
Avoidance of Public Eating					Learn to eat 3 proper meals a day.
Meal Skippers					Learn to eat 3 proper meals a day. Understand that proper eating does not lead to weight gain.
The Grazer					Learn to eat 3 proper meals a day. Eliminate all snacks.
The Sweet Tooth					Limit sugars to special occasions. Use sugar-free alternatives. Find alternate forms of reward.
Liquid Calories					Ideally, switch to plain water. Use sugar-free alternates.
Comfort Eating					Treat any underlying depression. Stress management. Avoid eating out of entitlement. Find alternate forms of reward.
Binge Eating					Stress management. See: Comfort Eating.
Dieting					Get off the diet wheel-spinning. Start recognizing the power of normal eating!
Eating out of Boredom/Eating to Stay Awake					Select labor-intensive, low calorie foods, chewing gum.

Severity Category
0 = Does not apply to me at all
1 = I have some of this kind of behavior
2 = This eating pattern plays a moderate role
3 = This is probably my main problem (or one of my main problems)

SIMON FENG, M.D.

EATING PATTERNS SELF-ANALYSIS CHART (Follow-up)

Date Completed: _____

Unhealthy Eating Pattern	Severity Category 0	1	2	3	Suggested Action
Non-Waster of Food					Leave food uneaten at every meal. Do not equate food with money.
Food as Entertainment					Enjoy **quality** of food, not **quantity**. Find alternate forms of reward. Avoid "Macho" eating.
Avoidance of Public Eating					Learn to eat 3 proper meals a day.
Meal Skippers					Learn to eat 3 proper meals a day. Understand that proper eating does not lead to weight gain.
The Grazer					Learn to eat 3 proper meals a day. Eliminate all snacks.
The Sweet Tooth					Limit sugars to special occasions. Use sugar-free alternatives. Find alternate forms of reward.
Liquid Calories					Ideally, switch to plain water. Use sugar-free alternates.
Comfort Eating					Treat any underlying depression. Stress management. Avoid eating out of entitlement. Find alternate forms of reward.
Binge Eating					Stress management. See: Comfort Eating.
Dieting					Get off the diet wheel-spinning. Start recognizing the power of normal eating!
Eating out of Boredom/Eating to Stay Awake					Select labor-intensive, low calorie foods, chewing gum.

Severity Category
0 = Does not apply to me at all
1 = I have some of this kind of behavior
2 = This eating pattern plays a moderate role
3 = This is probably my main problem (or one of my main problems)

SECTION FOUR

The New Approach

Chapter Eight: The Heterogeneous Nature of Obesity

"You can have it in any color you like, as long as it's black."
Henry Ford, when asked about choice of colors for the Model T Ford.

I believe that obesity is a heterogeneous condition. I think that people become obese for many different reasons and no single solution is going to be right for everyone. What I mean by the heterogeneous nature of obesity is that there are different kinds of obesity with different causes requiring different approaches and treatments. To understand heterogeneity, think of cars. You have 2-doors, 4-doors, hatch-backs, station wagons, SUV's and hybrids. You have domestics and imports, front-wheel drive, rear-wheel drive and all-wheel drive. You can't use the same tire on all those vehicles. I think of obesity like that. There are different causes of obesity that require different treatments. It is also not a case of "One Size Fits All".

> Different people are overweight for different reasons and the treatment cannot be a case of "One Size Fits All".

There isn't only one kind of overweight person. Overweight people differ in their expectations, in their motivations and in their resources. A slightly overweight 65 year old person, newly diagnosed with diabetes, has different motivation and expectations from an obese 25 year old single person wishing to lose 50 pounds for aesthetic reasons. The first person is far more interested in eating healthy, feels that the weight loss is do-able and essential, and may have a lifestyle that can accommodate the necessary changes. He or she may get the bulk of their extra calories from eating too much at meal times. The second person is more likely to feel that the goal is not really attainable; at the same time there is more impatience and a desire for quick results. He or she may get most of the extra calories between meals, snacking or drinking high calorie beverages. He or she may have a busier lifestyle that involves more stress, meals on the road, and more social pressures to attain a certain body-type. The younger person is also more likely to have a young family to cook for and healthy choices may be a little harder. The consequences of failure are not seen as impacting mortality.

My point is that these two people are not necessarily going to respond the same way to the same treatment plan.

Differences in Unhealthy Attitudes/ Unhealthy Eating Patterns

From the previous two chapters, I hope that it is obvious by now that different overweight people have different unhealthy attitudes and different unhealthy eating patterns. You cannot treat the Liquid Calorie overweight person in the same way that you treat the Comfort Eater. The differences among the various unhealthy eating patterns are by far the most important of the differences. There are also other differences that I would like to explore in this chapter.

Differences in Motivation

I have often noticed that one of the groups most likely to succeed in permanent weight loss is the group who make a big change in their lifestyles out of concern for their health. Someone who has just been diagnosed with diabetes or someone who has just had a heart attack has some real motivation to get healthy. They have just had a serious wake-up call reminding them of their mortality. They may always have known that their weight is potentially detrimental to their health, but suddenly it is no longer only potential and it is no longer just a theory. It is sad that too often it takes a catastrophe before we are willing to take things seriously. I remember a patient who had tried every known way to quit smoking without success until he had a small heart attack. All of a sudden he quit cold turkey and has never gone back.

The question is: How do we make patients take their risk factors seriously before the major catastrophe? What I say here is applicable not just to weight loss but also to high cholesterol, high blood pressure and diabetes, as well as many other chronic diseases without a lot of symptoms. High cholesterol and high blood pressure especially are "silent killers" where the very first symptom may be a very serious event such as a heart attack, stroke or death.

The technique that I have found most successful in motivating my own patients to take their risk factors seriously is to compare their diseases with terrorism. I point out to my patients that an absence of symptoms cannot be safely ignored. America was feeling just fine on September 10, 2001. The economy was good, there was a big surplus in the Treasury, and most people were about to get a healthy tax refund. The Cold War was over and America was at peace. The world was a different place the next day. Terrorists had hijacked two commercial airliners and flown them into the Twin Towers of the World Trade Center in New York City. Another commercial jet had been hijacked and crashed deliberately into the Pentagon. A fourth hijacked airliner crashed into a field without hitting its intended target due to the bravery and sacrifice of the passengers on board. Thousands died in America.

How and why did we let this happen? It wasn't that we did not know the Twin Towers were targets for terrorists; terrorists had tried to blow up the World Trade Center Towers once before in 1993 with a car bomb but did not inflict any structural damage. It wasn't because we did not realize that airline security was not adequate. The security company responsible for airport security had been cited on many previous occasions. It most certainly was not because we did not know about Osama bin Laden. We knew that he had orchestrated the bombings of two American embassies in Africa and the bombing of the USS Cole. Hollywood had made numerous movies about terrorists attacking office buildings and other similar scenarios. Even though we knew all of these, they were not real. They were things that happened to other people in other parts of the world.

What have we learned? Hopefully we have learned that the absence of symptoms doesn't mean squat. If we know that there are terrorists in the country, we must take action. If we know that we have high cholesterol or diabetes, we cannot afford to wait until we wake up in the Coronary Care Unit of our local hospital with tubes coming out of every orifice before we act.

Obesity is such a big risk factor for so many diseases that we must act before we find out that we are diabetic or have some other serious health problems. Some of the diseases known to be worsened by obesity include,

1. type 2 Diabetes mellitus
2. hypertension

3. coronary heart disease
4. congestive heart failure
5. dysmetabolic syndrome
6. dyslipidemias (high cholesterol /low good cholesterol)
7. osteoarthritis
8. sleep apnea
9. certain cancers (prostate, breast, colon, endometrial)
10. depression
11. gallstones

Motivation is really important when you wish to make a significant lifestyle change, and understanding the consequences of inaction is often helpful in getting the proper motivation. Do not forget the lesson of 9-11.

Differences in Expectations

Different patients can have very different expectations for a weight loss program. Generally, the younger the patient, the more important it is to have an aesthetic improvement, whereas the older patients care less about aesthetics and much more about their health and quality of life.

If you have an overweight married couple about 60 years of age or so, happily married for 35 years, looking sexy is not their prime motivation. Undoubtedly, they would not mind looking slimmer but what they really care about is to be able to move around better, in less pain, on fewer medications, and be able to do more things. It actually means something to these people if you tell them that a weight loss of 10 or 15 pounds would be very beneficial.

On the other hand, 25 year old single people hoping to attract a mate usually have aesthetic improvement as their most important objective. They expect to fit into a smaller clothing size, look more attractive and get more compliments. If you tell these people that a small weight loss of 10 pounds can still have a very significant health benefit, they instantly tune out and feel that whatever you have to say to them is not relevant to them.

If you feel that certain parts of this book do not apply to you, you're probably absolutely right!

Differences in Patience Level

Younger patients wishing to lose a significant amount of weight to look and feel better generally want significant results, fast! People wishing to lose weight for health reasons tend to be more willing to wait for more gradual weight loss. They understand that their health problems will continue to improve with gradual weight loss.

There is actually an important difference between this difference in patience and the above differences in expectations. The above-mentioned differences in expectations are all valid. Expecting to lose a lot of weight very quickly is neither reasonable nor healthy. The faster the weight loss the less likely it is to be permanent.

Differences in Resources

By differences in resources, I do not necessarily mean financial resources, although this may also play a role. I also mean social resources and emotional resources.

A divorced single mother of 3 kids, all under the age of 6, simply cannot be expected to have a meaningful exercise program. Just getting enough sleep is a serious challenge; let us not insist that she partake in an hour of moderate exercise every day. It was also for people like this that I stated back in Chapter One that exercise should not be considered mandatory for weight loss but just strongly recommended.

Social resources can also be a big factor. Having supportive friends and relatives can be helpful. Sometimes, however, it is a very negative factor. I have a patient who is the only overweight person in her family. She is often compared to her older sister who is slim, better looking and naturally athletic.

SIMON FENG, M.D.

Differences in Biology

I also emphasize that people come in different shapes and sizes. The ideal weight for a St. Bernard and a Greyhound are very different even though both breeds of dog are similar in height and length. Similarly, I believe that people also are built differently. If you ever get a big man like a NFL linebacker and get him to look like a marathon runner, you have a sick man on your hands. Similarly, there is no way under the sun that you could get a pole-vaulter to look like a professional wrestler. Instead, I like to concentrate on being healthy and eating normally. You will end up weighing exactly what you should be weighing. Your "Ideal Body Weight", which some medical charts give you, may not be the same as the weight that is the healthiest for you.

> People come in all different shapes and sizes. Your "Ideal Body Weight" may not be the same as the weight that is the healthiest for you.

Many people who are mildly overweight but not obese may be at their proper weight. This is not always an easy thing to tell them as they still wish to look like the glamorous models on the cover of magazines. Make sure that you are healthy and fit, eat properly, and you will end up where your healthy weight should be. Also, I suspect that at least for some people, a small weight gain of 5 to 10 pounds in middle age may not be "abnormal".

Differences in Confidence

I have had many patients who announced to me on the day I diagnosed them to be diabetic, "I will lose the necessary weight." They know before they start that they will succeed.

Other people have very little confidence. They may have tried all kinds of diets before without long-term success. They may feel a certain degree of hopelessness. They do not dare to try a new weight loss program because in their minds, they have already failed it. It is far easier for them to resign themselves to a lifetime of being fat than to take the risk of failing again.

FENG'S WAY: TO PERMANENT WEIGHT LOSS

Take heart! I am not asking for another diet. I am just asking for you to eat normally and think normally about food. Surely there is no risk in that?

Chapter Nine: Childhood Obesity

"There is no such thing as other people's children." – Hillary Rodham Clinton

Stemming the Epidemic

The most important aspect of dealing with any epidemic is to contain the spread of the disease. In dealing with the epidemic of obesity the emphasis on containment or prevention should similarly take precedence. We need to find a way to stop the next generation from developing the same unhealthy attitudes toward food that put them at risk of obesity.

As I discussed earlier, a "One Size Fits All" approach just doesn't work. This is especially true for the child or adolescent. It is fairly obvious that an obese 15-year old needs to be treated differently from an overweight 7-year old.

Basic Principles

1. From the statistics showing the epidemic of obesity, we must assume that *all* children are potentially at some risk of obesity, even if their parents are not overweight. Of course, children of overweight parents are probably at higher risk.

2. Older children need to be involved in their treatment. For the adolescent or teenager, it is definitely a case of "self-serve" medicine (Chapter Four), whereas younger children have less control of their food intake patterns.

3. We cannot be looking only at weight loss as children are growing. We also need to make sure that vertical growth is not compromised. This is especially a problem for traditional weight-loss diets, due to the fact that the child's nutrition may be compromised. However, because I am advocating a normal eating pattern, this should not be a problem.

SIMON FENG, M.D.

Nevertheless, the child's growth should be monitored by his/her doctor or health care provider.

4. Childhood depression must be identified and treated. Depression in children does not necessarily follow the same symptoms as adults. Please keep in mind that all too often, teenage depression goes unrecognized by the parents until some tragedy strikes.

Prevention

Prevention means making sure that our children do not develop the unhealthy attitudes responsible for abnormal weight gain. We need to make sure we do not instill any compunction to eat everything offered to them on a plate.

A limit must be put on sodas and sugar snacks. While adolescents have some access to these treats directly, younger children do not and their access must be limited. Just as people cannot become addicted to cigarettes unless they have access to cigarettes, kids cannot become "addicted" to sugar unless they have access to it. Often, parents switch from sodas to sports drinks or fruit juices, not aware that the sugar contents of these can be every bit as high as with sodas. Water is best but diet soda for older kids may be a good alternative.

I am not suggesting that children should never be allowed sweet treats but merely that their access be limited. Children will go out on Halloween night and come back with their loot. Allow them three days of these treats, after which you should make the treats disappear, permanently. They should not feel deprived. I fail to see why they need to be eating Halloween candy three weeks later. Kids have always wanted, and will always want sugar. Talk to your parents and grandparents and they will tell you that they enjoyed sugar as children. I know that I did. However, wanting sugar doesn't mean that we have to give them unlimited sugar! They will not love you less if you do not always give in to them.

I believe that in many instances, we give our children sweets to make up for our own feelings of inadequacy. Working parents may feel bad about having to put their children into daycare, and so find it difficult to refuse giving them sweets.

After-school snacks are okay but must be limited. Offer healthier alternatives such as grapes or yogurt. Even a small bag of potato chips is probably alright if the child has only one or two snacks a day; however, never allow the child to eat mindlessly while watching TV. When children snack, they should do so in the kitchen and they should not be doing anything else at the time. If children fall into the habit of sitting in front of a TV set with a big bag of chips every day, they are headed for trouble. If kids are snacking while they are watching TV or reading, or otherwise mentally engaged in some other activity, they are really not paying attention to their snack. I call this "Mindless Eating". They don't really need to eat but do so merely out of habit. Mindless eating is very much like smoking; you do it automatically even when you aren't really enjoying it. Just like smoking, it can be stopped. Once stopped for a few months, it is usually not even missed.

> Avoid "Mindless Eating".

We must not use sugar as a reward system. We certainly do not want to reward finishing the food on their plate (overeating) with dessert. Do not reward good behavior with candy. Buy trading cards for them, or take them to the park, the zoo, or to a movie. If you get popcorn at the movie theater, get a small size only.

We must never encourage our children to continue to eat after they are no longer hungry. Even if _we_ do not feel that they have eaten enough, do not insist that they keep eating! Many parents become very concerned if their children do not eat well for a few days. If the child does not wish to eat much at one particular meal or for one day, they may be compensating for overeating at a previous meal. If they are not hungry, there is little reason to make them eat. Do not worry - children have a lot of reserve capacity. When children are sick and unable to eat well for a week, they bounce back very quickly once able to eat again. It takes weeks if not months of chronic poor nutrition before the _normal_ child's health is seriously affected. Also, with many toddlers, it is not unusual for the child to eat well two or three days a week and not so well the other four or five days. Do not be concerned about malnutrition unless they are not growing well. Make sure the children get regular check-ups, measuring their heights and weights. If there is any concern with the child's growth, his or her doctor or health care provider should be able to advise you.

> Do not be concerned about malnutrition unless they are not growing well.

Do not instill guilt in them for "wasting" food and do not associate "wasting food" with "wasting money".

Never make overeating a "macho" thing for boys. It is not a smart thing to eat a 48 oz porterhouse in one sitting, and we must not praise boys for being able to eat a large amount of food. If they think of themselves as people who can "eat a ton", can weight problems be far behind? Let us teach our children to enjoy the quality of food rather than the quantity of food.

A hundred years ago, we used to think of skinny kids as being "sickly". Mothers also used to take pride in raising fat babies and fat children, feeling that this signified their superior homemaking skills. Presumably, they were such good cooks their kids all became overweight. Unfortunately, many people still think so. Let us arrive at the 21st century. We have much better measures of the child's health than the weight alone. Today, overweight children are far more likely to be in poor health than their thinner classmates. As they grow older, the negative effects of their weight only get worse. We know that overweight children are more likely to have self-esteem issues as well as suffer from depression. Overweight children grow up into overweight adults with even more health problems. If you want to give your child the gift of good health, do not make them overeat! Do not worry that your child is looking "sickly". Better to have a child whose weight is in the 15th percentile for his/her height than in the 75th percentile. If you are really concerned, have your child checked by your doctor or health care provider and let them tell you if the child is unhealthy.

> "Skinny" kids are not the same thing as "sickly" kids. If you wish to give your children the gift of good health, do not make them overeat!

Be very careful what kind of body image ideal we instill into our children. If kids think they need to look a certain way they are more likely to develop unhealthy eating patterns. Do not teach our children to diet.

Treatment

If a child is already overweight, treatment must depend on the age of the child. The older the child, the more important it is that we involve the child. A fifteen year old must wish to lose weight or it will not work. Teenagers as a group have little or no patience. If they hear that they will lose weight over the next year or so, they will not be pleased. They may not understand the concepts of permanent results. It is also "cool" for them to tell their peers that they are on a new diet, but telling their friends that they are starting to eat normally isn't as "cool" or exciting. On the other hand, if you tell them they can eat normally to lose weight, it might be well accepted. Teenage depression is also a big concern, especially because we know that overweight children are at more risk of depression.

All the above measures in the prevention of obesity should be implemented, as we must foster healthy eating. Otherwise, the treatment of obesity in children is similar to treatment in adults. We need to identify the unhealthy eating pattern(s) that may be at play and deal with them individually. Please refer again to Chapter Seven. We need to correct any unhealthy attitude towards food as well.

Exercise

An exercise program is always helpful. The problem is that the kids who are good in sports are not as likely to be overweight while the kids who would benefit most from exercise are likely not to enjoy sports as much. What many overweight children have a problem with is the competitive nature of sports in school. Overweight kids often do not feel that they can compete athletically with normal weight kids and so have little interest in sports. Get them involved in non-competitive sports not done in groups. Go throw a Frisbee with your kids. Get them one of those computer dance mats. Sign them up for martial arts. Weight training may be well accepted as well. *It works much better if you can make physical activity fun for the kids*

SIMON FENG, M.D.

rather than having a "no pain, no gain" mentality. Start slow and go slow. Overweight kids are not likely to be good at whatever physical activity it is you first introduce them to, but will get better with time.

Ideally, get the children to exercise without making it "exercise". If it is a fun activity for them, like dancing or throwing a Frisbee, they can get a workout without the feeling that it is like a chore or homework. Try to avoid letting the kids develop negative connotations about exercise.

> Overweight kids often do not feel that they can compete athletically with normal weight kids and so have little interest in sports.

Especially for the younger children, exercise can be encouraged with little effort. Limit their time in front of the TV and they may automatically become more active. Young children naturally equate physical activity as fun. Watch any kindergarten class at recess if you have any doubts on this score. Observe the games they play at recess and try to reproduce them in the evenings and on weekends.

Child Obesity Prevention and Treatment Questionnaire

Below is a questionnaire that is presented in chart form to allow you to see at a glance what areas may need attention. Besides this chart, if the child is already overweight, you will also need to go through the Eating Patterns Self-Analysis Charts at the end of Chapter Seven.

Child Obesity Prevention and Treatment Questionnaire

	Yes/No	Recommended Action
Could your child be depressed? (remember that it is not always recognized)		It is very important to treat child depression. Get them in with a child psychiatrist.
Does your child consume soda regularly?		Limit sodas to special occasions. Use diet sodas only if absolutely necessary.
Do you use sugar as a reward?		Find and cultivate other reward systems.
Does your child snack mindlessly?		This must stop. It is not easy but can be done.
Do you encourage your child to finish his or her plate?		Do not associate uneaten food as waste of either food or money. Do not make them eat after they are full.
Do you praise your child for being able to eat a lot?		Do not make overeating a point of self-esteem.
Does your child have a history of dieting?		Discuss unrealistic body image issues. Stop dieting and start eating normally.

Other Directions for the Future

The above suggestions only work on an individual-by-individual basis. This approach, by itself, can slow down but is unlikely to solve the epidemic of obesity. To deal with the obesity epidemic issue, we need more of a Public Health approach. I feel that education is going to be crucial. We have had many successes in the past century with other public health issues. For example, mass immunizations have made many diseases, such as pertussis, once common (it used to be the number one killer of children under the age of two), now rare in America. Pap smears and mammograms have put a big dent in

SIMON FENG, M.D.

cervical and breast cancers. Better dental hygiene has also greatly improved our general dental health.

Perhaps what we really need is to have a new discipline that I think of as "Interventional Sociology". More than likely what we also need is to educate the child through the educational system and the parents through public health programs or Ad campaigns. Popular magazines may play a role. Possibly we need to be teaching our children about unhealthy eating patterns along with dental hygiene. Somehow, we need to stop the epidemic!

Chapter Ten: The Game Plan

"So many of our dreams seem impossible, then improbable, then inevitable." – Christopher Reeve

The Content of Our Food

Up to this point, I have not discussed much about the fat content in our diet versus the carbohydrate content or the protein component. If you are waiting for recipes, I am going to disappoint you as well. I am only going to talk in generalities. My main goal is to get people to think and eat like normal weight people. Normal people do not go through their normal lives dissecting the content of their diet into carbohydrate and fat components. Neither should you.

This is not to say that it doesn't matter what you eat. On the contrary, it means a great deal. Sugar and fatty foods need to be curtailed but not by counting how many grams of fat are on your plate. You "simply" need to correct your attitudes toward food and eat for the right reasons. Most snacks are eaten for the wrong reasons and need to be eliminated. On the other hand, if you get really hungry and it is another hour before suppertime, go ahead and grab a light snack, just like any normal weight person would do.

I have not mentioned very much about the fat and cholesterol in our diets. My emphasis in this book has been on why we eat rather than on the contents of what we eat. Please understand that I definitely do encourage that you follow a low cholesterol, low fat diet for the sake of your heart, whether or not you are overweight. The biggest reason that I do not say too much about the contents of our diet is because I want to avoid turning this into another diet book, preaching what you can't eat. I am not giving anyone free license to eat whatever they want.

Try to make healthier choices in the food you select. Concentrate on eating a well-balanced diet with lots of vegetables. I know that some of you will be making faces at the thought of eating lots of vegetables. Part of the problem may be that you are accustomed to

SIMON FENG, M.D.

high fat foods and fried foods; you are not used to healthy foods. Give it a chance - in time you will find that you actually enjoy salads and other healthier foods. Don't make it a diet! Do not eat salads for the sake of losing weight but for the sake of eating healthy. You may need to acclimatize to your new way of eating.

I explain acclimatization in this way: if I were to wake you up at 3:00 am and turn on your bed-side lamp with a 40 watt bulb, the light will be blinding and painfully bright. Fifteen minutes later, you will realize that 40 watts is really very dim. It just seemed bright because you were not used to it. Eating healthy is like that but unfortunately takes more than 15 minutes to get used to. Eat healthy everyday for two or three months and I guarantee that you won't go back.

The Need for Vitamins

Many weight loss programs recommend vitamins and nutritional supplements. The biggest reason for this is that patients on their weight loss programs are not eating normally. They are eating less food and may not get enough vitamins and minerals. My game plan is for people to eat normally; therefore, vitamin supplements may not be as necessary or essential. Go ahead and take a multi-vitamin if you wish. My personal advice is not to spend a lot of money on vitamins and nutritional supplements. Do not let anyone scare you into taking vitamins. Remember the adage, "Believe half of what you see and nothing of what you hear." Ask yourself if the person giving you all this advice on vitamins stands to benefit from your buying them.

I remain of the thought that if you eat normally, there is unlikely to be a big need for vitamin supplements in most healthy people. Folic acid supplementation may not be a bad idea as it may reduce some people's heart disease risks and also helps to prevent some types of birth defects if taken early in pregnancy. I won't argue with some extra vitamin C although I do not think mega doses are necessary. Extra calcium is probably helpful for some people. There are also times when we use vitamins to treat specific medical problems but for the normal healthy person, vitamin deficiency is just not a big problem. At no time in the history of mankind has any group of human beings enjoyed better nutrition than Americans today. As long as you have a good varied diet, vitamin deficiency should not be an issue. If you have a very restrictive diet, such as if you were a vegetarian, it may make more sense to take some supplements. Still, if it will make you feel better, go ahead and take a multi-vitamin. As for bioflavinoids, co-enzyme Q-10's, or other supplements, I refer you back to Chapter Three.

The Role of Bariatric Surgery, Revisited

I am very fond of telling my patients that, "Nothing that we do for you as doctors is really good for you. It is not good to be taking pills, letting someone cut your belly open with a scalpel, putting your arm in a cast, sticking needles into your arm or shooting X-rays at you. We only do these things when it is better that we do them than we do not do them." If you are having a lot of trouble breathing and coughing up blood, I doubt that many would object to us taking X-rays, sticking IV needles into your arm and giving you medicine. Similarly, if your appendix was about to rupture, I really think it is a good idea for us to be cutting into your abdomen to take it out.

> Nothing that we do for you as doctors is really good for you. We only do things when it is better that we do them than we do not do them.

It is only in this light that I ever recommend bariatric surgery. As a clear example, let us suppose that you have a horrendous family history where both of your parents and all 4 of your older siblings had diabetes and all died of heart attacks before the age of 48 and you are just turning 45. You weigh 294 pounds and stand only 5 foot 7 inches tall. It may not be unreasonable to try some of the interventions we discussed in this book, but I think it is definitely worthwhile to consider bariatric surgery. I would tell a patient like this, "If you were to see six other people walk ahead of you down a dark alley and all six were mugged, beaten up and killed, for Pete's sake find a different way to go wherever it is you have to go! At the very least, do not go down the same alley without an armed escort!" Bariatric surgery may be drastic but at least you have a chance. To do nothing is madness.

Your own case may not be so desperate. What I wanted to illustrate in the hypothetical case above is that sometimes there is a real sense of urgency, and under those circumstances bariatric surgery may be considered first-line treatment.

The other time you really need to consider bariatric surgery is when nothing else works. I have mentioned that sometimes the causes of obesity are too deeply entrenched or the psychological background is too severe. If the interventions mentioned in this book are unable to help you, it may also be time to consider surgery.

The Role of Diets and Weight Loss Programs, Revisited

I have mentioned on more than one occasion that obesity is a very heterogeneous condition and that different people may need very different approaches. There are many people who definitely benefit from a very structured weight loss program or diet plan.

If this describes you, you may be happy to know that my approach to permanent weight loss may be compatible with many other weight loss programs! Weight loss programs, managed meal plans, low calorie diets and low carbohydrate diets all deal with caloric imbalance. I am convinced that working on the caloric imbalance alone is not sufficient and we really need to be working on the underlying reasons why the caloric imbalance exists. However, this approach does not preclude tackling the caloric imbalance directly as well. There may certainly be many advantages to trying to correct the "what" we eat at the same time that we are working on the "why" and "how" we eat.

Feng's Way to Permanent Weight Loss can be compatible with many weight loss programs.

There are however, some notes of caution.

1. Do not fall into the "diet mentality" where food becomes the most important thing in your life. I have stated that I consider dieting to be an unhealthy eating pattern. This is mostly because of the "diet mentality". If you can avoid this mentality and try to normalize your attitudes toward food as well as the way you eat, being conscious of what you eat is definitely a good thing.

2. Address your unhealthy attitudes toward food. I believe that the people who succeed long-term at weight loss through diet plans also changed their attitudes toward food.

3. Do not expect a permanent result from a temporary change. If you expect to lose weight on a diet and keep the weight off, you also need to make some sort of a permanent change. I have stated that diets can help you to lose weight but are not as effective at keeping the weight off. People who lose weight on a diet and manage to keep the weight off long-term have either corrected the underlying unhealthy attitudes and eating patterns or have adopted a new "Dietary Way of Life". For a diet to work long-term, the diet should not be a form of deprivation.

4. Stick to three meals a day with minimal snacking (preferably none at all). Learn to eat to the point of comfort rather than to the point of discomfort. Normalize your eating.

If you concentrate on trying to correct your attitudes toward food and getting rid of your unhealthy eating patterns, you should find that results should be much easier to maintain.

Feng's Way, The Game Plan

We have covered a lot of information so far in this book and hopefully you agree with some or most of my assertions. What I would like to do now is to summarize briefly the main principles in this book and organize it into a game plan. The method of weight loss that I advocate is undoubtedly very different from what most people are used to thinking of as necessary for weight loss. They may still feel that I should be giving them a list of prohibitions of what they cannot be eating. I feel very strongly that the treatment of obesity must be directed not so much at **what** people eat but at **how** and **why** they eat. I believe that when people learn to get rid of their unhealthy eating patterns, they automatically reduce the calories that they consume, which will result in the desired weight loss.

> When people learn to get rid of their unhealthy eating patterns, they automatically reduce the calories that they consume, which will result in the desired weight loss.

Make no mistake about it, this Game Plan that I suggest may not be simple. It is rather complicated and you may need to put in some real effort, but the results are worth it. I offer a new approach that can give you permanent results that does not require surgery or long term medications, and that the weight loss need not be a life-long battle to maintain. However, I never claimed that it was going to be easy. Most worthwhile things in life require effort and some perseverance, be it a successful marriage, a good job, good parenting or a university degree. Every time I see or hear an advertisement for weight loss products or programs, there is always a claim that it is easy. "Lose 20 pounds in 3 easy steps!" or "Four easy weeks to a healthier, slimmer you!" or some other similar headline. There is the perception that weight loss should be easy. With my approach, some people may find it easy. For example, someone whose excess calories all come from soda pops might find the change quick and easy. Others for whom the abnormal eating patterns comprise a mixed bag of different reasons may find it quite difficult. Bad habits are not always easy to break, but generally with the right motivation it can be done.

Back in Chapter Four, I described the concept that the treatment of some diseases is a full-service treatment but other diseases required a self-service approach. The non-surgical treatment of obesity requires a self-service approach. It does require commitment and real effort. Will power does not really enter into this because I am only trying to change your mental attitudes toward food. I believe that if you can successfully change your attitude toward food into a normal one, weight loss will become automatic and even inevitable.

Below are the steps that I suggest in my game plan:

1. **Rule out medical problems**
   Make sure that you don't have hypothyroidism or other medical reasons for weight gain. Address these problems if they are present. If you have to be on some medical diet such as a diabetic diet, this takes precedence. You can still follow many of

the principles of this book such as not cleaning off your plate every meal, addressing comfort-eating issues and so on, but stay on your prescribed diet. Similarly, if you have been told to follow a low cholesterol diet, you can still follow the principles in this book but be aware of what you are eating and make better choices on the foods you eat, selecting low fat foods.

2. **If there is urgency, consider proceeding directly to bariatric surgery**
   If you have significant health issues or feel that your comfort eating is secondary to psychological reasons that are too deeply entrenched, this might not be unreasonable. However, almost always, at least a short trial of the modifications I suggest in this book should be tried first.

3. **Identify the unhealthy eating patterns, identify the sources of the extra calories**
   Go through the sections of unhealthy attitudes and eating patterns. Figure out which one(s) apply to you. Fill out the Eating Patterns Self-Analysis Chart. Understand your own unhealthy attitudes.

   Decide on whether you want to make all the changes at the same time or take on one change at a time. My preference would be to make all changes together as it is often easier to make a complete change then continue little battles for a long time. Think of spring cleaning – it may be much more efficient to take one day to clean the whole house all at once, rather than to clean one room at a time, only to have the clean rooms messy again before you get to the last room. However, I also recognize that people are different and may prefer to do things differently.

4. **Normalize your eating habits!**
   As mentioned at the end of Chapter Seven, concentrate on:
   a. enjoying three good meals a day
   b. learning not to overeat at mealtimes
   c. minimizing snacks

5. **Concentrate on permanent results**
   With any change that you consider making, be sure that they are changes you will be able to keep up forever. Concentrate on normalizing your attitudes toward food. Do not make this about

your weight but concentrate on eating like a normal person. Think and eat like a normal weight person, never like a fat person trying to lose weight. Do not have a target weight.

6. **Institute an exercise program**
The importance of this cannot be overstated. Make the focus of the exercise improving your health and fitness. You will find that with exercise, you will enjoy how you feel, you will experience more energy. You can enjoy little achievements such as being able to run up a flight of stairs without feeling tired. You will feel younger! All these positive things will occur if you keep up an exercise program for even a month or so. The positives will encourage your continuing participation with or without weight loss. Even if you cannot lose weight, it is far better to be fit and overweight than unfit and overweight. You will enjoy better health.

Throughout this book you will notice that I believe we need to follow a normal lifestyle. Before the sociological changes I talked about in Chapter Six, and before the advent of all those wonderful labor-saving devices, exercise was an unavoidable part daily living. Don't worry; I am not suggesting that you give up cars and washing machines. However, you do need to recognize that we are less active nowadays, so we need to institute an exercise program to balance our more sedentary lifestyles. I mention this because if you are not used to a formal exercise program, it does not feel like a natural or normal thing to do. I know that not every normal weight person exercises regularly (although as a medical doctor I recommend it) and although I do think it is possible to lose weight without exercising, I still think exercise is very helpful.

7. **Eat healthy**
Change the content of your food to a healthier one. Learn to eliminate junk food not because you are trying to lose weight but because it does not fit in with your new healthy attitudes and eating patterns.

8. **Have reasonable expectations**
- Remember that different people have different body types. Some people are "bigger boned" than others and will always weigh more than someone else the same height. Fat *distribution* is often genetically determined. If you have thick

ankles and wrists because your parents had thick ankles and wrists, do not expect this to respond to any degree of weight loss.
- Keep in mind that the slower the weight loss, the more likely that the weight loss will be permanent.
- If after you normalize your life and your attitudes, you find that you have lost weight but still end up several pounds heavier than you would like, this is may be your healthy weight.
- It is okay to feel hungry. Normal people without weight problems feel hungry at mealtimes. Slight hunger is normal. Remember the thirst model: treat your hunger like thirst - it's not a catastrophe. When you are thirsty, you drink something (it doesn't have to be soda-pop) until you quench your thirst but you do not drink two gallons at one sitting, hide in a closet to drink, or drink non-stop for the whole day. Do not eat in these unhealthy ways either.

> Treat hunger the way you treat thirst.

9. If you can't lose weight

If you do not succeed in weight loss with my model, do not despair. Try to determine if:
- your failure is because you have not identified all the unhealthy eating patterns, or
- it is due to the fact that you have been unable to correct the unhealthy eating patterns that you have identified.

If you have not succeeded in making the necessary changes but continue to feel that my socio-cultural model makes sense, try again after a few weeks. Knowing what to change and being able to make the change happen is not the same thing. Everyone who smokes today realizes that he or she should quit, but not everyone has quit. I would like to point out that far more people succeed in quitting smoking than in losing weight permanently. I would also like to point out that most people who succeeded at smoking cessation did not manage to quit on the very first attempt but only after several attempts.

Perhaps you need to get some professional help by way of counseling or seeing your doctor/health care provider about possible depression. Also, make sure he or she rules out any medical reasons for weight gain.

Perhaps you may not have identified all the unhealthy eating patterns that may be at work in you. Re-read the book and see if you do not fit into a different category of unhealthy eating, or to make sure you haven't swapped one unhealthy pattern for another in the process of making changes in your attitude toward food.

I am not trying to be pessimistic but realistic in realizing that my methods will not help everybody lose weight. What I would like is for people to get off the merry-go-round of diets, appetite-suppressants and herbal weight loss, and recognize that those do not work long term.

> Most people who succeeded at smoking cessation succeed only after several attempts. If you do not succeed in weight loss with my model, try again after a few weeks.

10. If nothing works
At this time, if your health is *seriously threatened* by your weight problem, you really should consider bariatric surgery.

Final Thoughts

In this book I have tried to develop some of my ideas about weight loss. This is what makes sense to me and my hope is that it makes sense to you too. I started out wanting to write a short essay but as my ideas developed and my thoughts gelled, I found that my model of weight problems and obesity quickly gained in complexity. I began to realize that the various different types of unhealthy eating patterns overlapped to a large degree. I have attempted to make this book more user-friendly by providing charts for you to personalize your particular unhealthy eating pattern so that you can figure out what you need to change.

My goal is to have people finally understand what it was that made them gain weight in the first place. There is an ancient

Chinese philosopher, Sun Tzu, who said "To guarantee victory, you need to know yourself and know your enemy." I am convinced that people who count calories and go on diets know neither themselves nor their enemy.

Just as some people need help to quit smoking, there may be many people who understand and agree with what I say but cannot succeed by themselves. Self-help books can only go so far. The people most helped are the ones with considerable insight and are honest with themselves. Sometimes the same principles work better when applied by a professional instead of in a self-help setting. Perhaps the future will see weight loss clinics using these principles to help those unable to make the necessary changes on their own accord. Hopefully this book will find acceptance among health care providers who will be willing and able to help. I feel sure that the abnormal eating patterns I describe are real. I hope other professionals, be they dietitians, therapists, sociologists or physicians, may join me in refining my ideas and treatments.

APPENDIX

REFERENCES

GLOSSARY

INDEX

Appendix

Body Mass Index (BMI) Charts

Body Mass Index, or BMI, is a measure of body weight and height which is useful to reflect how fat a person is. It allows us to compare a 6 foot tall man with a 5 foot tall woman. It is defined as a person's weight in kilograms divided by the square of their weight in kilograms.

$$BMI = \frac{\text{Weight in kilograms}}{\text{Height in meters)}^2} \quad \text{or} \quad \frac{\text{Weight in pounds} \times 703}{\text{(Height in inches)}^2}$$

In general, a BMI of less than 25 is considered to be normal. BMI's of 25 to 30 fall into the overweight category. Obesity is defined as a BMI of greater than 30 but is further classified into Class 1 with BMI of 30 to 35, Class 2 with BMI of 35 to 40, and Class 3 or morbid obesity with a BMI of greater than 40.

BMI	Classification
<25	Normal
25 – 30	Overweight
30 – 35	Class 1 Obesity
35 – 40	Class 2 Obesity
>40	Class 3 Obesity (morbid obesity)

The BMI is meant only as a guide as you will notice that it does not measure the percentage of body fat. Because of this, it is really hard to apply the BMI guidelines to athletes. A person's BMI may be high because he or she has too much fat but also the BMI may be high if the person has too much muscle bulk. An obvious example is the professional body-builder who may have extremely low body fat but still have a BMI in the obese category.

It is also to be noted that different ethnicities have different degrees of percentage body fat for the same BMI. At the same BMI

SIMON FENG, M.D.

level, Asians are "fatter" than Caucasians, who in turn are "fatter" than African Americans. In other words, an Asian with a BMI of 23 may be "fatter" than an African American with a BMI of 26.

BMI TABLE

	WEIGHT IN POUNDS										
		120	130	140	150	160	170	180	190	200	210	220
HEIGHT IN FEET AND INCHES	4'5"	30	33	35	38	40	43	45	48	50	53	55
	4'6"	29	31	34	36	38	41	43	46	48	51	53
	4'7"	28	30	33	35	37	40	42	44	47	49	51
	4'8"	27	29	31	34	36	38	40	43	45	47	49
	4'9"	26	28	30	33	35	37	39	41	43	46	48
	4'10"	25	27	29	31	34	36	38	40	42	44	46
	4'11"	24	26	28	30	32	34	36	38	40	43	45
	5'0"	23	25	27	29	31	33	35	37	39	41	43
	5'1"	23	25	27	28	30	32	34	36	38	40	42
	5'2"	22	24	26	27	29	31	33	35	37	38	40
	5'3"	21	23	25	27	28	30	32	34	36	37	39
	5'4"	21	22	24	26	28	29	31	33	34	36	38
	5'5"	20	22	23	25	27	28	30	32	33	35	37
	5'6"	19	21	23	24	26	27	29	31	32	34	36
	5'7"	19	20	22	24	25	27	28	30	31	33	35
	5'8"	18	20	21	23	24	26	27	29	30	32	34
	5'9"	18	19	21	22	24	25	27	28	30	31	33
	5'10"	17	19	20	22	23	24	26	27	29	30	32
	5'11"	17	18	20	21	22	24	25	27	28	29	31
	6'0"	16	18	19	20	22	23	24	26	27	29	30
	6'1"	16	17	19	20	21	22	24	25	26	28	29
	6'2"	15	17	18	19	21	22	23	24	26	27	28
	6'3"	15	16	18	19	20	21	23	24	25	26	28
	6'4"	15	16	17	18	20	21	22	23	24	26	27
	6'5"	14	15	17	18	19	20	21	23	24	25	26
	6'6"	14	15	16	17	19	20	21	22	23	24	25
	6'7"	14	15	16	17	18	19	20	21	23	24	25
	6'8"	13	14	15	17	18	19	20	21	22	23	24
	6'9"	13	14	15	16	17	18	19	20	21	23	24
	6'10"	13	14	15	16	17	18	19	20	21	22	23

BMI TABLE

	WEIGHT IN POUNDS										
		230	240	250	260	270	280	290	300	310	320	330
HEIGHT IN FEET AND INCHES	4'5"	58	60	63	65	68	70	73	75	78	80	83
	4'6"	56	58	60	63	65	68	70	72	75	77	80
	4'7"	54	56	58	61	63	65	68	70	72	75	77
	4'8"	52	54	56	58	61	63	65	67	70	72	74
	4'9"	50	52	54	56	59	61	63	65	67	69	72
	4'10"	48	50	52	54	57	59	61	63	65	67	69
	4'11"	47	49	51	53	55	57	59	61	63	65	67
	5'0"	45	47	49	51	53	55	57	59	61	63	65
	5'1"	44	45	47	49	51	53	55	57	59	61	62
	5'2"	42	44	46	48	49	51	53	55	57	59	60
	5'3"	41	43	44	46	48	50	51	53	55	57	59
	5'4"	40	41	43	45	46	48	50	52	53	55	57
	5'5"	38	40	42	43	45	47	48	50	52	53	55
	5'6"	37	39	40	42	44	45	47	49	50	52	53
	5'7"	36	38	39	41	42	44	46	47	49	50	52
	5'8"	35	37	38	40	41	43	44	46	47	49	50
	5'9"	34	36	37	38	40	41	43	44	46	47	49
	5'10"	33	35	36	37	39	40	42	43	45	46	47
	5'11"	32	34	35	36	38	39	41	42	43	45	46
	6'0"	31	33	34	35	37	38	39	41	42	43	45
	6'1"	30	32	33	34	36	37	38	40	41	42	44
	6'2"	30	31	32	33	35	36	37	39	40	41	42
	6'3"	29	30	31	33	34	35	36	38	39	40	41
	6'4"	28	29	30	32	33	34	35	37	38	39	40
	6'5"	27	29	30	31	32	33	34	36	37	38	39
	6'6"	27	28	29	30	31	32	34	35	36	37	38
	6'7"	26	27	28	29	30	32	33	34	35	36	37
	6'8"	25	26	28	29	30	31	32	33	34	35	36
	6'9"	25	26	27	28	29	30	31	32	33	34	35
	6'10"	24	25	26	27	28	29	30	31	32	34	35

References

Epidemic of Obesity

Allison DB et al. Annual deaths attributable to obesity in the United States. Journal of the American Medical Association 1999; 282(16): 1530-8

Flegal KM et al. Prevalence and Trends in Obesity Among US Adults, 1999-2000. Journal of the American Medical Association 2002; 288(14):1723-27

> The increases in the prevalence of obesity and overweight previously observed continued in 1999-2000.

Freedman DA et al. Trends and correlates of Class 3 obesity in the United States from 1990 through 2000. Journal of the American Medical Association 2002; 288(14): 1758-61

> This very important study followed the prevalence of morbid obesity and showed the differences by race and educational achievement level.

Mokdad AH et al. The spread of the obesity epidemic in the United States, 1991-1998. Journal of the American Medical Association 1999; 282(16): 1519-22

Mokdad AH et al. The continuing epidemics of obesity and diabetes in the United States. Journal of the American Medical Association 2001; 286(10): 1195-1200

Mokdad AH et al. Prevalence of obesity, diabetes, and obesity-related health risk factors, 2001. Journal of the American Medical Association 2003; 289 (1): 76-9

> These 3 articles by Mokdad et al are the source of the maps of the prevalence of obesity presented in Chapter Two.

Must A et al. The disease burden associated with overweight and obesity. Journal of the American Medical Association 1999; 282(16): 1523-9

Ogden CL et al. Prevalence and Trends in Overweight Among US Children and Adolescents, 1999-2000. Journal of the American Medical Association 2002; 288(14):1728-32

SIMON FENG, M.D.

The prevalence of overweight and children in the US is continuing to increase, especially among Mexican-American and non-Hispanic black adolescents.

Troiano RP et al. Overweight prevalence and trends for children and adolescents: The National Health and Nutrition Examination Surveys, 1963-1991. Archives of Pediatric and Adolescent Medicine 1995; 149: 1085-91

Prevalence of overweight in children has been increasing from 1963-1991

Genetics of Obesity

Bray MS et al. OB gene not linked to human obesity in Mexican American affected sib pairs from Starr County, Texas. Human Genetics 1996; 98(5): 590-5

Carlson B et al. Obese (ob) gene defects are rare in human obesity. Obesity Research 1997; 5(1): 30-5

Costanzo PR, Schiffman SS. Thinness—not obesity—has a genetic component. Neuroscience Biobehavioral Reviews 1989; 13(1):55-8

Comparing adopted children with their birth parents and adoptive parents showed that genetics did not play a significant role in obesity

Esparza J et al. Daily energy expenditure in Mexican and USA Pima Indians: low physical activity as a possible cause of obesity. International Journal of Obesity and Related Metabolic Disorders 2000;24(1):55-9

Price RA et al. Obesity in Pima Indians: large increases among post World War II birth cohorts. American Journal of Physical Anthropology 1993; 92(4): 473-9

Pima Indians did not become obese until after WW II

Ravussin E et al. Effects of a traditional lifestyle on obesity in Pima Indians. Diabetes Care 1994; 17(9): 1067-74

Pima Indians in Mexico had an average BMI of 24.9 compared to 33.4 for USA Pima Indians. Diabetes rates among Mexican Pima Indians were 11% in women and 6% in men compared to USA Pima Indian rates of 37% and 54% respectively.

Health Effects of Obesity

Allison DB et al. Annual deaths attributable to obesity in the United States. Journal of the American Medical Association 1999; 282(16):1530-8

Allison DB, Saunders SE. Obesity in North America, an overview. The Medical Clinics of North America 2000; 84(2): 305-32

Dixon JB et al. Depression in association with severe obesity – changes with weight loss. Archives of Internal Medicine 2003; 163: 2058-65

Klein S. Outcome success in obesity. Obesity Research 2001; 9(4)S: 354-8

Must A et al. The disease burden associated with overweight and obesity. Journal of the American Medical Association 1999; 282(16): 1523-9

Herbal Remedies

FDA Consumer Advisory, June 6, 2003. Vinarol and Viga tablets contaminated with Sildenafil (viagra) FDA safety alerts at www.fda.gov/medwatch/SAFETY/2003/safety03.htm

> Author's note: Most of the information regarding the safety and efficacy of herbal remedies are not readily available except from the manufacturer's websites. The nature of the herbal/nutritional supplement industry is best revealed in investigative reports rather than scientific journals.

Consumer Reports. November 1995 "Herbal Roulette" pages 698-705

> An older article but still good.

Ellen Shell "One Can Make You Small" in O The Oprah Magazine, August 2003, pp146-149,181

> Excellently done piece of investigative journalism.

Low-Carbohydrate Diets

Bravata DM et al. Efficacy and safety of low-carbohydrate diets. Journal of the American Medical Association 2003; 289(14):1837-50

> This study looked at data collected for 3268 patients. Weight loss while using low carbohydrate diets was principally associated with

decreased caloric intake and increased diet duration but not with reduced carbohydrate content.

Appetite Suppressants

Connolly HM et al. Valvular heart disease associated with fenfluramine-phenteramine. New England Journal of Medicine 1997; 337:581

> This was the first article that pointed to an association between taking fen-phen and heart valve abnormalities.

Jick H et al. A population-based study of appetite-suppressants drugs and the risk of cardiac-valve regurgitation. New England Journal of Medicine 1998; 339:719

Khan MA et al. The prevalence of cardiac valve insufficiency assessed by trans-thoracic echocardiography in obese patients treated with appetite-suppressant drugs. New England Journal of Medicine 1998; 339:713

National Task Force on the Prevention and Treatment of Obesity. Long-term pharmacotherapy in the management of obesity. Journal of the American Medical Association 1996; 276(23): 1907-15

> Weight loss tends to plateau after 6 months and some studies show partial weight regain despite continued drug therapy.

Weissman NJ et al. An assessment of heart-valve abnormalities in obese patients taking dexfenfluramine, sustained-release dexfenfluramine, or placebo. New England Journal of Medicine 1998; 339:725

Bariatric Surgery

Balsiger BM et al. Bariatric Surgery – surgery for weight control in patients with morbid obesity. The Medical Clinics of North America 2000; 84(2): 477-89

Brolin RE. Bariatric surgery and long term control of morbid obesity. Journal of the American Medical Association 2002; 288(22): 2793-6

Cottam DR et al. Laparoscopic era of operations for morbid obesity. Archives of Surgery 2003; 136: 367-75

Livingston EH, Aaron AS. Quality of life – cost and future of bariatric surgery. Archives of Surgery 2003; 136: 383-8

Mason EE. Development and future of gastroplasties for morbid obesity. Archives of Surgery 2003; 138:361

Long Term Weight Loss

Ayyad C, Anderson T. Long-term efficacy of dietary treatment of obesity: a systematic review of studies published between 1931 and 1999. Obesity Reviews 2000; 1(2): 113-9

Donnelly JE et al. Effects of a 16-month randomized controlled exercise trial on body weight and composition in young, overweight men and women: the Midwest Exercise Trial. Archives of Internal Medicine 2003; 163(11): 1343-50

Klem ML et al. A case control study of successful maintenance of a substantial weight loss: individuals who lost weight through surgery versus those who lost weight through non-surgical means. International Journal of Obesity and Related Metabolic Disorders 2000; 24(5): 573-9

National Task Force on the Prevention and Treatment of Obesity. Long-term pharmacotherapy in the management of obesity. Journal of the American Medical Association 1996; 276(23): 1907-15

Ogden J. The correlates of long-term weight loss: a group comparison study of obesity. International Journal of Obesity and Related Metabolic Disorders 2000; 24(8): 1018-25

Sheperd TM. Effective management of obesity. Journal of Family Practice 2003; 52(1)

Wing RR, Hill JO. Successful weight loss maintenance. Annual Reviews in Nutrition 2001; 21:323-41

> Successful long term weight loss maintainers (defined as losing 10% or more of initial weight and keeping the weight off for 1 year or more) were found to share certain characteristics such as eating less fat, frequent weight monitoring and high level of physical activity.

Differences Between Obese and Normal Weight

Becker ES et al. Obesity and mental illness in a representative sample of young women. International Journal of Obesity and Related Metabolic Disorders 2001; 25 suppl 1:S5-9

SIMON FENG, M.D.

> In young women, obesity is related to increased rates of mental disorders, most notably anxiety disorders.

Everson SA et al. Epidemiological evidence for the relation between socioeconomic status and depression, obesity, and diabetes. Journal of Psychosomatic Research 2002; 53(4): 891-5

> Data from 4 large epidemiological studies on the role of psychological characteristics, social factors, and behaviors in health and disease risk.

Goodman E et al. Adolescents' perceptions of social status: development and evaluation of a new indicator. Pediatrics 2001; 108(2): E31

> Subjective social status and psychological health related to risk of obesity.

Hulshof KF et al. Socioeconomic status, dietary intake and 10 year trends. European Journal of Clinical Nutrition 2003; 57(1):128-37

> Prevalence of obesity and skipping of breakfast was higher among people of low socioeconomic status (SES).

Ortega RM et al. Differences in the breakfast habits of overweight/obese and normal weight schoolchildren. International Journal of Vitamin and Nutrition Research 1998; 68(2):125-32

> Overweight children had poorer breakfast habits than normal weight children.

Ortega RM et al. Associations between obesity, breakfast-time food habits and intake of energy and nutrients in a group of elderly Madrid residents. Journal of the American College of Nutrition 1996; 15(1): 65-72

> Normal weight subjects ate more for breakfast, had more variety and took longer to eat breakfast compared to overweight subjects.

Sociological Aspects of Obesity

Ball K, Mishra G, Crawford D. Which aspects of socioeconomic status are related to obesity among men and women? International Journal of Obesity and Related Metabolic Disorders 2002; 26(4):559-65

> Low status employed women were 1.4 times more likely to be overweight than high status employed women.

Freedman DA et al. Trends and correlates of Class 3 obesity in the United States from 1990 through 2000. Journal of the American Medical Association 2002; 288(14): 1758-61

Frenn M et al. Addressing health disparities in middle school students' nutrition and exercise. Journal of Community Health Nursing 2003; 20(1):1-14
> Those of low income, esp. African American and Hispanics, have the greatest risk of inactivity and obesity.

Hulshof KF et al. Socioeconomic status, dietary intake and 10 year trends. European Journal of Clinical Nutrition 2003; 57(1):128-37
> Prevalence of obesity and skipping of breakfast was higher among people of low socioeconomic status (SES).

Jeffery RW, Rick AM. Cross-sectional and longitudinal associations between body mass index and marriage-related factors. Obesity Research 2002; 10(8): 809-15
> Husbands and wives tend to share similar BMI's probably due to similarities in eating patterns.

Kaluski DN et al. Overweight, stature and socioeconomic status among women – cause or effect? Journal of Gender Specific Medicine 2001; 4(4):18-24
> The level of one's education and one's stature were significantly, independently associated with BMI. Low stature and obesity were indicators of low educational attainment.

Reidpath DD et al. An ecological study of the relationship between social and environmental determinants of obesity. Health & Place 2002; 8(2):141-5
> Relationship between an area measure of SES and the density of fast-food outlets was examined. It was found that there was a dose-response between SES and the density of fast-food outlets. People living in areas of lowest SES had 2.5 times the exposure to outlets than people in the wealthiest category.

Sobal J, Stunkard A. Socioeconomic status and obesity: A review of the literature. Psychology Bulletin 1989; 105: 260-75
> In developed countries there is an inverse relation between socioeconomic status and obesity.

Wang J et al. Asians have lower body mass index but higher percent body fat than do whites: comparisons of anthropometric measurements. American Journal of Clinical Nutrition 1994; 60:23-8
> BMI may not mean the same thing in different races.

Wang J et al. Comparisons for body mass index and body fat percent among Puerto Ricans, blacks, whites and Asians living in the New York City area. Obesity Research 1996; 4:377-84
> BMI may not mean the same thing in different races.

Wang Y. Cross-national comparison of childhood obesity: the epidemic and the relationship between obesity and socioeconomic status. International Journal of Epidemiology 2001; 30(5): 1129-36

> Child obesity is becoming a public health problem worldwide, but the prevalence of obesity varies remarkably across countries with different socioeconomic development levels.

Wardle J et al. Sex differences in the association of socioeconomic status with obesity. American Journal of Public Health 2002; 92(8): 1299-304

Dieting as an Unhealthy Eating Pattern

Birch LL, Fisher JO. Mothers' child-feeding practices influence daughters' eating and weight. American Journal of Clinical Nutrition 2000; 71: 1054-61

Birch LL, Fisher JO Development of eating behaviors among children and adolescents. Pediatrics 1998; 101: 539-49

Johnson SL, Birch LL. Parents' and children's adiposity and eating style. Pediatrics 1994; 94(5): 653-61

Childhood Obesity

Anderson PM, Butcher KF, Levine PB. Maternal employment and overweight children. Journal of Health Economics 2003; 22(3):477-504

> Child is more likely to be overweight if his/her mother worked more hours per week over the child's life. Higher socioeconomic status mothers' work intensity particularly deleterious for children's overweight status.

Birch LL, Fisher JO. Mothers' child-feeding practices influence daughters' eating and weight. American Journal of Clinical Nutrition 2000; 71: 1054-61

Brewis A. Biocultural aspects of obesity in young Mexicans. American Journal of Human Biology 2003; 15(3):446-60

> More likely to be obese if boys from small households with few or no other children and more permissive, less authoritarian parents.

Goodman E et al. Adolescents' perception of social status: development and evaluation of a new indicator. Pediatrics 2001; 108(2)

Robinson TM et al. Is parental control over children's eating associated with childhood obesity? Results from a population-based sample of third graders. Obesity Research 2001; 9(5): 306-12

Troiano RP et al. Overweight prevalence and trends for children and adolescents: The National Health and Nutrition Examination Surveys, 1963-1991. Archives of Pediatric and Adolescent Medicine 1995; 149: 1085-91

> Prevalence of overweight in children has been increasing from 1963-1991

Wang Y. Cross-national comparison of childhood obesity: the epidemic and the relationship between obesity and socioeconomic status. International Journal of Epidemiology 2001; 30(5): 1129-36

> Child obesity is becoming a public health problem worldwide, but the prevalence of obesity varies remarkably across countries with different socioeconomic development levels.

Author's Note: The above studies at least suggest the possibilities of childhood obesity being correlated with sociological issues such as socioeconomic status, parental supervision and parenting styles. Of note, the incidence of childhood obesity in China has increased very significantly possibly due to an increase in prosperity and the "One Family One Child" policy in China causing a more permissive parenting style.

Glossary

A

aesthetics the philosophy or the theory of beauty.
adverse effects in pharmacology and therapeutics, an undesired side-effect or toxicity caused by the administration of drugs.
allergic reaction n. a reaction in which the body becomes hypersensitive to a particular chemical and results in either local or general effects, varying from asthma to dermatitis and occasionally circulatory collapse.
anatomy n. the study of the form and gross structure of the various parts of the human body.
anorexia nervosa a psychological illness in which patients starve themselves or use other techniques, such as vomiting or taking laxatives in order to induce weight loss
appetite suppressants chemicals or medications taken to induce weight loss by reducing appetite.
atropine n. a drug extracted from deadly nightshade (see belladonna) that inhibits the action of certain nerves of the autonomic nervous system.

B

bariatrics n. the field of medicine concerned with the study of obesity – its causes, prevention and treatment.
bariatric surgery the field of surgery concerned with the surgical treatment of obesity.
Belladonna n. deadly nightshade (*Atropa belladonna*); the plant from which the alkaloids belladonna, atropine, and hyoscyamine are obtained.
beta-blockers a drug that prevents stimulation of the beta-adrenergic receptors of the nerves of the sympathetic nervous system and therefore decreases the activity of the heart.
blind loop syndromes a condition of stasis of the small intestine allowing for overgrowth of bacteria which causes mal-absorption and the passage of fatty stool.

BMI (Body Mass Index) also called *Quetelet's index*, which is derived by dividing one's weight (in kilograms) by the square of one's height (in meters). In pounds and inches, you need to multiply the result by 703. BMI is used in the definition of overweight and obesity.
botulism n. a serious form of food poisoning from foods containing the toxin botulin produced by the bacterium Clostridium botulinum.
bulimia a psychological illness of insatiable overeating often ending in self-induced vomiting. May be a phase of anorexia nervosa.
by-pass n. a surgical procedure to divert the flow of blood or other fluid from one anatomical structure to another; a shunt (in the case of gastric bypass, food is diverted from the stomach to the small bowel much further downstream)

C

CFC chlorofluorocarbon. Any of various compounds consisting of carbon, hydrogen, chlorine and fluorine, once widely used as aerosol propellants and refrigerants. CFC's are believed to cause depletion of the atmospheric ozone layer
calorie n. a unit used to indicate the energy value of foods which is equal to the amount of heat required to raise one kilogram of water from $14.5°C$ to $15.5°C$.
carbohydrates n. a large group of compounds including sugars and starch that contain carbon, hydrogen and oxygen. Carbohydrates are an important source of energy: they are manufactured by plants and obtained by animals and man through the diet, being one of the three main constituents of food other than fat and protein.
carcinogenic adj. the property of any compound that, when exposed to living tissue may cause the production of cancer.
cardiac conditioning improving the physical capability of the heart by an exercise program
causality n. the relation of cause and effect.
conventional medicine the practice of medicine according to standards generally accepted by practitioners graduating from accredited universities and licensed by the State.
Cushing's syndrome the condition arising from an excess of corticosteroid hormone in the body. Symptoms include weight gain, reddening of the face and neck, excess growth of body and facial hair, raised blood pressure, loss of mineral from the bones, raised glucose levels and sometimes mental disturbances.

D

DHEA dehydroepiandrosterone (also called GL701, prasterone), a hormone secreted from the adrenal gland with androgenic (or male hormone) activity.
diet n. 1. the mixture of foods that a person eats. 2. a prescribed course of eating and drinking in which the amount and kind of food are regulated for a therapeutic purpose.
digitalis n. an extract from the dried leaves of foxglove (Digitalis species), which contains various substances including digitoxin and digoxin which stimulate heart muscle. Used to treat heart failure.
diuretic n. an agent that increases urine secretion
double-blind a method of scientific investigation in which neither the subject nor the investigator knows what treatment, if any, the subject is receiving.
dumping syndrome a syndrome marked by sweating and weakness after eating, occurring in patients who have had gastric resections.
dyslipidemia a condition of abnormal cholesterols or triglycerides.
dysmetabolic syndrome a syndrome marked by obesity, high blood pressure, diabetes and high cholesterol, putting the patient at much higher risk of cardiovascular disease. (also called metabolic syndrome and syndrome X)

E

echinacea a herbal product that is used to treat a variety of common ailments from the common cold and psoriasis. Also called black susans, black Sampson, braunia sp., Indian head, purple cone flower, etc.
ephedra a herbal medication with amphetamine-like activity used in the treatment of asthma, bronchitis and as an appetite suppressant. Also called ma-huang, sea grape, herbal ectasy, desert herb, popotillo, yellow astringent and yellow horse.
epidemiology the study of the distribution and determinants of health-related states and events in populations, and the application of this study to the control of health problems.
estrogen any natural or synthetic substance that induces estrus and the development of female sexual characteristics; more specifically, the estrogenic hormones produced by the ovary; the female sex hormones.

F

FDA the Food and Drug Administration. In the US, an official regulatory body for foods, drugs, cosmetics, and medical devices. It is part of the US Department of Health and Human Services.
feverfew an herbal medication used to treat headaches, migraines, menstrual irregularities, fevers, arthritis, allergies, psoriasis, tinnitus and vertigo. Also known by a host of other names.

G

gastric stapling a form of bariatric surgery where a large portion of the stomach is isolated from the rest of the organ by a band of staples.
gluten enteropathy also called celiac sprue; a disease of the small intestine marked by intolerance and mal-absorption of a type of protein known as gluten.
growth hormone a hormone secreted by the anterior pituitary gland that regulates the cell division and protein synthesis necessary for normal growth.

H

herb n. a plant with a soft stem containing little wood, esp. an aromatic plant used in medicine or seasoning.
heterogeneous of unlike natures; composed of unlike substances.
hormone n. a substance originating in an organ, gland or body part that is conveyed through the blood to another body part, chemically stimulating that part to increase or decrease functional activity or to increase or decrease secretion of another hormone.
hydrophilic the property of a chemical that has affinity for water.
hypothyroidism n. sub-normal activity of the thyroid gland, causing mental and physical slowing, undue sensitivity to cold, slowing of the pulse, weight gain, and coarsening of the skin.

I

ideal body weight Ideal body weight formulas were derived from the Metropolitan Life Insurance Company height and weight tables

L

laxatives n. a food or chemical substance that acts to loosen the bowels (ie. Facilitate the passage of bowel contents at the time of defecation) and therefore prevent constipation
lipophilic the property of a chemical that has an affinity for fat.
liposuction the surgical removal of subcutaneous fat tissue with a blunt tipped cannula introduced through a small incision. It is a plastic surgery procedure done for aesthetic reasons.

M

ma-huang see ephedra
mal-absorption disordered or inadequate absorption of nutrients from the intestinal tract.
mal-nutrition disorder of nutrition causing a lack of necessary or proper food substances in the body
melatonin a hormone produced in the pineal gland. It may be involved in the onset of puberty and may influence wake-sleep cycles.
metabolism the sum of all physical and chemical changes that take place in the body; all energy and material transformations that take place within living cells.
metabolism boosters (thermogenic agents) natural or chemical agents that speed up the metabolic rate, or the rate of using up energy.
metastatic cancer spread of cancer beyond its original location to distant parts of the body
morbid obesity also called Class 3 obesity, defined as having a BMI of over 40. This class is associated with the highest health risks from obesity.

N

nutitional supplements vitamins and minerals used to supplement the diet.

O

obesity defined as a BMI of over 30

P

perforation n. the process of a hole forming in an organ
phytoestrogen n. a chemical of plant origin having female sex hormone activity
placebo n. an inactive substance given to a patient; used in the controlled study of drugs
placebo-controlled adj. a type of scientific method of study where the control group does not get any active medicine.
prednisone a glucocorticoid with the same effect as cortisone
prevalence the number of cases of a disease in a specified population at a given time
proprietary belonging to a proprietor or owner of a product or brand name. Exact make-up of compounded formulas need not be disclosed.

Q

quantum a fixed unit or amount of material not usually further sub-divided.

R

RDA recommended daily allowance: the amount of vitamins and/or minerals suggested to prevent deficiency.

S

satiety the state of being full to satisfaction (of food)
saw palmetto an herbal product used most often for the treatment of prostate enlargement.
sedentary lifestyle a lifestyle involving little exercise
sociology the science or study of the origin, development, organization and functioning of human society
standardized to bring to or make of an established standard size, weight, quality strength or the like.

T

testosterone a male sex steroid hormone secreted by the testes, promoting the growth of secondary male sexual characteristics
toxicity the poisonous effect of a substance

U

UNICEF an agency of the United Nations charged with improving the health and nutrition of children and their mothers throughout the world. (United Nations International Children's Emergency Fund)

V

Vitamins any of a group of organic substances other than proteins carbohydrates, fats and organic salts that are essential for normal metabolism, growth and development of the body.

Index

A

acclimatization · 130
acupuncture · 32
adrenal glands · 51
aesthetic improvement · 116
alcoholism · 12, 25, 45
allergies · 27
all-you-can-eat buffet · 69
anatomy · 4, 47, 48
antabuse · 43
anti-depressants · 7, 53, 54
appetite suppressants · 4, 42
arthritis · 36, 39, 53, 56, 57
aspirin · 27
atropine · 27, 157
authoritarian parenting · 72

B

bariatric surgery · 4, 7, 12, 47, 48, 95, 131, 132, 135, 138
binging · 98, 99
biochemistry of satiety · 40
blind-loops · 47
body-image · 99
botulism toxin · 26
breakfast · 68, 76, 77, 88, 91, 152, 153

C

caloric imbalance · xi, 46, 61, 62
calorie counting · 74
cancers · 26, 116
carbohydrates · 7, 8, 88, 100, 158
cardiac conditioning · 39
central obesity · 51
chemical imbalance · 53
chewing gum · 100
childbirth · 32, 52, 72
childhood obesity · 22, 154, 155
chronic fatigue · 53
cocaine · 26
comfort eating · 53, 70, 71, 87, 94, 95, 96, 98, 99, 135
confidence · 33, 118
congestive heart failure · 116
Cushing's syndrome · 33, 40, 43, 52, 159
cystic fibrosis · 44

D

definition of obesity · xii
depression · 35, 39, 40, 51, 52, 53, 56, 90, 96, 152
DHEA · 35, 159
diabetes · 15, 16, 35, 39, 40, 41, 48, 52, 86, 94, 113, 114, 115, 131, 147, 152
diabetic diet · 134
diet mentality · 10, 73
Dietary Way of Life · 9
dietitians · 49, 70, 139
digitalis · 27, 159
diuretics · 37
dumping syndromes · 47, 48
dyslipidemia · 159
dysmetabolic syndrome · 116, 159

E

eating in public · 87, 88
eating out of boredom · 101
Echinacea · 27, 159
education · 73, 153
enjoyment of food · 76, 85, 87
entitlement · 69, 70, 95, 96
ephedra · 27, 32, 38, 159
evidence-based medicine · 36
exercise · xiv, 6, 10, 11, 12, 21, 46, 96, 117, 125, 126, 136, 151, 153, 158, 163

F

fatigue · 51, 53, 54
feelings of inadequacy · 71
Fenfluramine · 42
Fen-Phen · 42
fertilizers · 28
fibromyalgia · 53
Food and Drug Administration · 25
food as a surrogate for love · 71
food as reward · 86, 95
food critics · 85
foxglove · 27
full-service · 41, 43, 48, 134

G

gallstones · 116
genetic · xii, 43, 44, 45, 46, 69
ghrelins · 40
gingko · 29
ginseng · 29
ginsenoside · 30
grazing · 72, 88

H

heart attack · 9, 16, 39, 114
herbicides · 28
high blood pressure · 12, 15, 40, 42, 52, 54, 114
Hippocratic Oath · 25
hormones · 35, 40, 44, 46
hypertension · 46, 115
hypothyroidism · 5, 40, 43, 51, 57, 134, 161

I

Ideal Body Weight · 118
immediate gratification · 95
insecticides · 28
insulin sensitivity · 44
irritable bowel syndrome · 53

J

junk foods · 10, 70

L

Law of Conservation of Energy · 5, 6, 7, 13
laxatives · 37
leptins · 40
lipase-inhibitors · 42
low cholesterol diet · 135
low-carbohydrate diets · 7, 8, 74, 100, 149

M

mal-absorption · 47, 48, 161
malnutrition · 10, 48, 88
Marilyn Monroe · 65
masculine prowess · 72
meal-skipping · 99
medications that cause weight gain · 55
melatonin · 35, 161
metabolism boosters · 4, 37
migraine headaches · 27, 54
minerals · 10, 88, 130
Miss America pageant · 65
morbid obesity · 48, 143, 150, 151, 162

N

neurotransmitters · 53
nicotine patches · 55
Nutrasweet · 92

O

obesity · xii, xiv, 8, 13, 39, 40, 46, 47, 48, 49, 51, 61, 62, 63, 66, 67, 72, 73, 75, 76, 113, 121, 138
Osama bin Laden · 115

osteoarthritis · 116

P

pathological attitudes · 62, 69, 73, 76, 79, 99, 100, 114, 121
pathological eating patterns · 7, 52, 55, 56, 65, 76, 79, 87, 99, 103, 114, 135, 138
peanut allergies · 27
permissive parenting · 72, 73, 155
pesticides · 28
Phenteramine · 42
phytoestrogens · 28, 162
poor self-esteem · xii, 39, 95, 98, 99
portion sizes · 68, 93
post-partum depression · 52
poverty · 67
prednisone · 7, 32
pregnancy · 52
preparation of food · 72
prevalence · 44, 63, 147, 148, 154, 155
prevalence of obesity · 15
prevention of obesity · 79
processed foods · 63
propranolol · 54
prosperity · 63, 67, 155
psychotherapy · 87, 95, 96

Q

quantumization of food · 68

R

rationalize inappropriate eating · 96
RDA (recommended daily allowance) · 77
role models · 65, 72

S

Saint Johns Wort · 29
SARS · 16
Saw Palmetto · 29
sedentary lifestyle · 39, 65
self-service · 41, 43, 134
sex-appeal · 65
sibutramine · 42
sickle cell disease · 44
skim milk · 93
sleep apnea · 54, 116
slow metabolism · 40, 51
smoking cessation · 56, 137, 138
socioeconomic strata · 67
sociology · 22, 61, 62, 163
soda-pop · 75, 92, 137
spinal cord injuries · 56
Splenda · 92
St. John's wort · 27
standard of beauty · 65
steroids · 51, 57
Steve Bechler · 27
stroke · 16, 31, 57, 114
structure of the family · 63
super-sizing · 68

T

Tang · 63
thermogenic agents · 37
time for preparation of meals · 63
tubocurare · 26
tumor necrosis factor-α · 40

U

unhealthy attitudes · 44, 69, 79, 122
unhealthy eating patterns · 52, 106, 125, 128
UNICEF · 82, 163

V

viagra · 33, 46, 149
vitamins · 10, 47, 77, 88, 130

W

wasting food · 67, 68, 100
West Nile Virus · 16
will power · 77, 134
willow bark · 27

wine critics · 85

Z

Zyban · 56

About the Author

Simon Feng was born in Taiwan and has spent his years living in many locations around the world including China, Malaysia, Canada and the United States. He received his Medical Degree from the University of British Columbia. He is certified by the College of Family Physicians of Canada. The author has practiced medicine in many different settings and varying locales, from the isolated rural mining town of Elkford in the Canadian Rockies to metropolitan downtown Toronto. (The town of Elkford is apparently the highest permanent settlement in Canada. Hence, his biggest claim to fame so far has been that, once upon a time, he was the "Highest Physician in the Land!") He is currently practicing Family Medicine in Johnson County, Indiana, and is on staff at Johnson Memorial Hospital in Franklin, Indiana. He resides with his family in Indianapolis.

Printed in the United States
16272LVS00004B/284-472